SMART HOME TECHNOLOGIES AND SERVICES FOR GERIATRIC REHABILITATION

SMART HOME TECHNOLOGIES AND SERVICES FOR GERIATRIC REHABILITATION

Edited by

MOHAMED-AMINE CHOUKOU

College of Rehabilitation Sciences; Centre on Aging, University of Manitoba, Winnipeg, Manitoba, Canada; Riverview Health Centre, Winnipeg, Manitoba, Canada

SHABBIR SYED-ABDUL

Graduate Institute of Biomedical Informatics, Adjunct Professor at School of Gerontology Health Management, Taipei Medical University, Taipei, Taiwan

ELSEVIER

ACADEMIC PRESS

An imprint of Elsevier

elsevier.com/books-and-journals

Academic Press is an imprint of Elsevier
125 London Wall, London EC2Y 5AS, United Kingdom
525 B Street, Suite 1650, San Diego, CA 92101, United States
50 Hampshire Street, 5th Floor, Cambridge, MA 02139, United States
The Boulevard, Langford Lane, Kidlington, Oxford OX5 1GB, United Kingdom

British Library Cataloguing-in-Publication Data
A catalogue record for this book is available from the British Library

Library of Congress Cataloging-in-Publication Data
A catalog record for this book is available from the Library of Congress

ISBN: 978-0-323-85173-2

For Information on all Academic Press publications visit our website at https://www.elsevier.com/books-and-journals

Publisher: Mara Conner
Acquisitions Editor: Sonnini R. Yura
Editorial Project Manager: Isabella C. Silva
Production Project Manager: Kamesh Ramajogi
Cover Designer: Christian J. Bilbow

Typeset by Aptara, New Delhi, India

Contents

7. From exergames to immersive virtual reality systems: serious games for supporting older adults

John E. Muñoz, Maria F. Montoya, Jennifer Boger

8. Big Data, Big Data Analytics application to Smart home technologies and services for geriatric rehabilitation

Matthew Willetts, Anthony S. Atkins, Clare Stanier

9. Conclusion and perspectives

Mohamed-Amine Choukou, Shabbir Syed-Abdul

Contributors

Alaa Abd-Alrazaq Division of Information and Computing Technology, College of Science and Engineering, Hamad Bin Khalifa University, Qatar Foundation, Doha, Qatar

Eiman Al-Jafar Health Informatics and Information Management, Faculty of Allied Health Sciences, Kuwait University, Kuwait

Dari Alhuwail Department of Information Science, College of Life Sciences, Kuwait University, Kuwait; Health Informatics Unit, Dasman Diabetes Institute, Kuwait

Majid H. Alsulami Department of Computer Science, Community College, Shaqra University, Shaqra, Saudi Arabia

Anthony S. Atkins School of Digital, Technologies and Art, Staffordshire University, Stoke-on-Trent, United Kingdom

Iman Azimi Department of Computing, University of Turku, Turku, Finland

Jennifer Boger Department of Systems Design and Engineering, University of Waterloo, Waterloo, Canada; Research Institute for Aging, Waterloo, Canada

Russell J. Campion School of Digital, Technologies and Art, Staffordshire University, Stoke-on-Trent, United Kingdom

Mohamed-Amine Choukou College of Rehabilitation Sciences; Centre on Aging, University of Manitoba, Winnipeg, Manitoba, Canada; Riverview Health Centre, Winnipeg, Manitoba, Canada

Enrique Dorronzoro-Zubiete Computer Engineering School, Universidad de Sevilla, Seville, Spain

K. Ganapathy Apollo Telemedicine Networking Foundation, Chennai, Tamil Nadu, India

Guido Giunti University of Oulu, Oulu, Finland; TU Delft, Delft, The Netherlands

Mowafa Househ Division of Information and Computing Technology, College of Science and Engineering, Hamad Bin Khalifa University, Qatar Foundation, Doha, Qatar

Riitta Mieronkoski Department of Nursing Science, University of Turku, Turku, Finland

Maria F. Montoya HCI Group, Universidad Tecnologica de Pereira, Colombia

John E. Muñoz Department of Systems Design and Engineering, University of Waterloo, Waterloo, Canada; HCI Group, Universidad Tecnologica de Pereira, Colombia

Thierry Oscar Department Of Drug Regulatory Affairs, RFW-University of Bonn, Germany

Laura-Maria Peltonen Department of Nursing Science, University of Turku, Turku, Finland

Octavio Rivera-Romero Computer Engineering School, Universidad de Sevilla, Seville, Spain; I3US: Research Institute of Computer Engineering, Universidad de Sevilla, Seville, Spain

Lydia Sequeira Institute of Health Policy, Management & Evaluation, University of Toronto, Toronto, ON, Canada; Centre for Addiction and Mental Health, Toronto, ON, Canada

José Luis Sevillano Computer Engineering School, Universidad de Sevilla, Seville, Spain; I3US: Research Institute of Computer Engineering, Universidad de Sevilla, Seville, Spain

Ali S. Sorour School of Digital, Technologies and Art, Staffordshire University, Stoke-on-Trent, United Kingdom

Clare Stanier School of Digital, Technologies and Art, Staffordshire University, Stoke-on-Trent, United Kingdom

Shabbir Syed-Abdul Graduate Institute of Biomedical Informatics, Adjunct Professor at School of Gerontology Health Management, Taipei Medical University, Taipei, Taiwan

Matthew Willetts School of Digital, Technologies and Art, Staffordshire University, Stoke-on-Trent, United Kingdom

List of reviewers

Dr. Carson K Leung, University of Manitoba, Canada

Dr. Eugene Loos, Utrecht University, Netherlands

Dr. Frank Knoefel, University of Ottawa, Canada

Dr. José Luis López Ruiz, Universidad de Jaén, Spain

Dr. Luis Fernandez-Luque, Salumedia Labs, Spain

Dr. Octavio Rivera, University of Seville, Spain

Dr. Oluwatoyin Sorinmade, Kent and Medway NHS and Social Care Partnership Trust, United Kingdom

Dr. Saleh Al Muayqali, Jouf University, Kingdom of Saudi Arabia

Dr. Yijin Wu, Qufu Normal University, Popular Republic of China

Preface

The increasing proportion of older adults requiring geriatric rehabilitation challenges the healthcare systems and the individuals, increasing levels of burden on the healthcare workers and the family members. There has been a growing interest in developing strategies to provide geriatric home care to decrease strain on geriatric facilities and increase the outcome of rehabilitation and the independence of the patients. Gerontechnologies have witnessed a boom over the last decade. In particular, smart home technologies and services pave the way for a new era of geriatric rehabilitation, supported by telemonitoring and tele-assistance services. Virtual reality platforms have gamified many interventions involving one or more "gamers" and are increasingly enabling the screening of cognitive impairments in apparently healthy older adults, such as declining memory. Moreover, thanks to telepresence robots and telemonitoring apps on smartphones and tablets, carers have never been closer to their beloved one. While these innovative solutions are available, many solutions are not implemented. Of the implemented interventions, there are still need to framework the modalities of modifying and measuring responses to rehabilitation interventions in geriatric populations. Acceptability, usability and adherence need further consideration. There are still plenty of technological problems to overcome. There is a strong need for society to set goals, address legal problems, policies, and regulations. In addition, business models need to evolve to keep up with the trend and meet priorities. Designed for a multidisciplinary audience, this book provides a toolbox for the design, development, and implementation of smart home solutions.

Acknowledgment

We dedicate this book to all advocates who seek to advance geriatric rehabilitation in order to empower seniors, their caregivers and health care providers, to researchers who offer new options for personalized care and new ways to enhance the capabilities of all stakeholders involved in seniors' health through ground-breaking digital technologies. We thank them for their commitment to transforming the rehabilitation sector to ensure access, equity, empowerment and patient participation. *"Smart Home Technologies and Services for Geriatric Rehabilitation"* was written with the participation of 26 authors from 12 countries: Canada, Columbia, Finland, Germany, India, Kuwait, Netherlands, Qatar, Saudi Arabia, Spain, Taiwan, and the United Kingdom. We thank them all for their time and dedication to the advancement of knowledge in geriatric rehabilitation.

CHAPTER

1

Geriatric Smart home technology implementation—are we really there?

K. Ganapathy

Apollo Telemedicine Networking Foundation, Chennai, Tamil Nadu, India

LEARNING OBJECTIVES

- The primary Learning Objective of this introductory chapter is for the reader to have a balanced view of the use of Smart Home Technologies (SHTs) for geriatric rehabilitation.
- Practical utilitarian value of SHTs from a clinician's perspective, demonstrating a clinical difference in healthcare outcomes is not the same as achieving technical success.
- Technology acceptance from the beneficiary's perspective is essential.
- Limitations, disadvantages, and the necessity to ensure that SHT is a tool and not an end by itself will be highlighted.

1.1 Introduction—geriatric landscape

"If I had known I was going to live this long, I would have taken better care of myself."—***Mae West***

"Smart *is not just a word; it is an attitude."*—***Ogwo David Emenike***

Though India centric, this introduction could be extrapolated to many other countries as well. The traditional joint family ecosystem prevalent in India for centuries is slowly disintegrating, exposing the vulnerability of elders. The author and his family were looking after his parents even when the latter were 84 and 94 years of age. Four generations living under one roof, in the authors' opinion was a win-win

Smart Home Technologies and Services for Geriatric Rehabilitation
DOI: https://doi.org/10.1016/B978-0-32-385173-2.00004-7

situation for everyone. There was an excellent quality of life for all. No one felt the absence of Smart homes and even the necessity for "rehabilitation." However, the world today is totally different. A report by the Confederation of Indian Industries (CII) suggested that India's elderly population will grow to 158 million by 2025. By the end of the century, seniors would constitute 34% of the total population. Ensuring adherence to minimum standards of safety and security for elders will require establishing and implementing quality and certification standards across elder care facilities. With increased regulatory and policy support from the government and investment from private sector entities, the senior care segment could emerge as a sunrise industry for India. The CII report points out that a specific legal and administrative policy is necessary [1]. India has around 100 million elderly at present. This may increase to 323 million by 2050, constituting 20% of the population. Among community dwelling residents, one-third over age of 65 and one-half over 80 may experience a fall each year. As of 2017, 92.4% of the elderly in India was physically mobile, implying that they could manage most of their day-to-day responsibilities. Only 5.5% were confined to their homes.

Money is not the only concern for India's elderly. A survey by HelpAge India estimates that 6% of senior citizens in India live alone. Loneliness is a problem that cuts across classes and is a challenge in cities as well. There are 10%–20% of senior citizens in India probably suffering from loneliness, a condition likely to be exacerbated by the current curbs on movement and contact due to the pandemic [2].People older than 65 years were more likely to share fake news in the United States. The situation in India could be similar with more than 200 million using WhatsApp for the primary source of new information, especially news. Misinformation and anxiety could be compounded during the pandemic [3]. An Agewell Foundation Study found about 85.8% of older adults in India were digitally illiterate. Studies however have shown that older adults are capable of acquiring digital literacy.

1.2 Background—aging elders their global distribution

Currently, 7% of the world's population is now over 65 years of age. The proportion of older people is expected to rise to 20% by 2050 [4,5]. In the European Union, 20% of population will be over 65 years of age by 2025 [6]. Compared to 2017, the number of persons aged 60 or older is expected to triple by 2100, rising from 962 million to 2.1 billion in 2050 and 3.1 billion in 2100. In Singapore alone those aged above 65 will double by 2030 to 900,000, accounting for 25% of the population [7]. Number of people aged over 85 (those most likely to require health and social care) will continue to rise. Between 2017 and 2040, the figure is estimated to increase from 1.4 to 2.7 million people. As per The Japan Times, 28% of Japanese are 65 years of age or older. By 2060, one in every 2.5 people will be 65 years or older. Following this trend, the elderly may comprise up to 38.4% of the population by 2065. Worldwide, by 2050 it is predicted that more people will be older than 60 years than under 15 years. Adults 85 and older in the United States will triple between 2015 and 2060—making it the fastest-growing age group over this time period. These statistics speak for themselves. Gerontology is here to stay.

1.3 Necessity for rehabilitation in the elderly

World Health Organization estimates that 15% of the world's population has some form of disability. Rehabilitation has a key role in decreasing level of disability. Application of advanced technologies in rehabilitation is a promising opportunity to attain this goal. In the last few decades, residential aged care facilities have been ensuring a safe friendly environment [8]. Setting meaningful, individualized rehabilitation goals is an essential part of the rehabilitation process [9]. New services, applications, and devices are being offered to prevent, compensate, care, and enhance daily life functioning of senior citizens Rehabilitation for impaired older adults is more effective and more fun [10]. A comprehensive geriatric assessment is necessary to individualize care for older adults [11]. The elderly have complex physical, cognitive, social, and emotional needs. Life expectancy of old people has increased. We also need to keep in mind that biological aging is not always a function of time. The prevalence of chronic, disabling diseases (cardiovascular diseases, diabetes mellitus, ophthalmological, neurological, locomotor, mental, chronic disorders, etc.) increases with aging.

1.4 Introduction to geriatric rehabilitation

Essential to geriatric rehabilitation is communication, specifically improving sensory impairment of vision and hearing. Prevention of falls and delaying osteoporosis can improve quality of life and longevity. Addressing malnutrition can promote healing and energize elders to participate in a formal rehabilitation program. Functional loss of mobility and inability to perform activities of daily living (ADLs) often lead to depression [12]. Assistive robots have been used to power wheelchairs, prosthetic limb controls, peripheral nervous systems, and home automation systems [13]. Technology readiness level for Smart homes and home health-monitoring technologies is low placement in a care facility, especially against an individual's wishes, and has been associated with depression, social isolation, and greater dependency in completion of self-care tasks. Older adults (almost 85%) prefer to obtain care in their homes rather than a healthcare institution [14]. Elderly, handicapped patients, and those with locomotion difficulties particularly when living alone can benefit from Smart homes [15]. Costs for elderly care range from $900 to over $5000 per month. Initial studies indicate that staying at home—or aging in place, as it is called—results in better health outcomes than moving to a care facility, especially when cognition and depression is the problem. Little attention has been paid to ethical challenges of Smart home applications for those approaching end of their lives.

1.5 Challenges in geriatric rehabilitation

Disability burden is related to number of coexisting chronic conditions. Poor performance occurs in all three disablement domains—body structure and function, activities, and participation. Multimorbidity compounds problems in rehabilitation [16]. Significant decrease in physical, cognitive, and sensory capabilities is an age-related phenomenon. Other influencing factors also cannot be accurately predicted as unexpected life events such as widowhood can make a difference. Smart home technology (SHT) is increasingly directed toward elders to enhance quality of life. Challenges, barriers, and beneficiary's acceptance of technology need to be considered. Including pleasurable experiences, which allows aging occupants to have fun while living in a Smart home and interacting with Smart devices, is a recent addition [17]. Informed consent is an ongoing process and not a single isolated event as decisions could change depending on initial experience, concerns regarding depersonalization, and introduction of new processes [18]. Sensorimotor rehabilitation forms an important part of the care provided after brain injury. This aims to restore loss of motor control and increase independence and quality of life. This is based on neural plasticity, the ability of the nervous system to reorganize its structure, function, and connections in response to training [19]. Understanding that plasticity is a fundamental property of the adult human brain, neuro-rehabilitation has taken a new meaning. Creating new neural pathways could be considered a disruptive technology [20]. A home for the elderly should offer peace, safety, security, and tranquility. Building a Smart home for elders requires involvement of licensed, skilled, and professional developers.

1.6 Technology acceptance by senior citizens

The technology acceptance model is an information systems theory that models how users *accept* and *use* a technology. The actual system use is the end-point where people use the technology. Behavioral intention is a factor that leads people to use the technology. This is influenced by the attitude, which is the general impression of the technology. When users are presented with a new technology, several factors influence their decision about how and when, they will use it. These include perceived usefulness—"the degree to which a person believes that using a particular aid would enhance his/her efficiency. Perceived ease-of-use is "the degree to which a person believes that using a particular system would be free from effort." If the technology is easy to use, then it is more accepted. External variables such as social influence are an important factor to determine the attitude. Perceptions are individualistic, depending on age, gender, circumstances, and time to device use. They included concerns about cost (42%) and a lack of familiarity with the technology (32%). Facilitators to device use included training prior to device use (61%) and tailoring devices to the functional needs of older adults (34%) [21]. mHealth devices and services are complex interventions that have to be integrated into an older person's life to facilitate effective use. People over 65 generally use fewer new technologies—including the Internet, smartphones, and other digital devices—and use them less frequently than younger people. Older, less educated, and less affluent people, as well as people with disabilities, appear to use them even less often [22]. Developers, providers, and policymakers should make sure that older people are included in decisions about technology use [23]. Transforming older adults into lead adopters of a new 24/7 lifestyle of being monitored, managed, and at times motivated, to maintain their health and wellness using technology is indeed a challenge [24]. Awareness of psychological and contextual factors is needed to facilitate aging in place through the use of technology [25]. Privacy can often be a barrier for older adults' adoption of Smart home IT [26]. Although an Internet-of-Things-based Smart home solution can provide an improved and better approach to healthcare management, yet its end user adoption is very low. Performance and effort expectancy, expert advice, and perceived trust are critical. Effort expectancy is the leading predictor of Smart homes for healthcare acceptance among the elderly [27].

1.7 Introduction to Smart homes

A Smart home is a convenient home setup where appliances and devices can be automatically controlled remotely with an Internet connection, using a mobile or other networked device [28]. Devices in a Smart home are interconnected through the Internet, allowing the user to control functions such as security access to the home, temperature, lighting, and a home theater remotely. The global home automation market was valued at about $53.5 billion by 2022. SHT for the elderly needs to specifically cover safety, health, physical activity, social engagement, and leisure.

Safety is about detecting and mitigating, if not removing, hazards from the user's environment. Social engagement relates to the Smart home functions that allow the elderly to combat social isolation, connecting the elderly with friends and family. Leisure activities are about how a Smart home can allow users to spend their free time. Technology-enabled physical activity relates to active engagement in Nonsedentary activities [29].

Smart locks, Smart lighting, apps, and gadgets for entertainment and communication, motion sensors and alerts, audio-enabled devices, medication reminders, and other technology-enabled wellness tools form a Smart home [30]. Smart locks can be programmed to grant access only to authorized personnel. Door cameras and Smart locks can be customized to allow individuals with mild impairments to be independent for longer. Smart homes increase domestic comfort, convenience, security, and leisure, reducing energy use through optimized home energy management. Automation, affordance, physical and psychological support promote independence. Acceptance is a key issue. Numerous initiatives worldwide have been developed to explore the use of motion sensors, radio frequency sensors, video cameras, wearable devices, and other applications that target older adults. The majority of the identified projects (71%) include technologies for functional monitoring (such as bed sensors, activity/motion sensors, and gait monitors). Water temperature sensors, stove sensors, and automatic light activation are examples.

Creating a connected home. Pressure-sensing floors, Smart furniture, and medical sensors, in addition to integrated appliances would require Smart devices to interpret context [31]. Older adults are likely to accept Smart-home technologies, if they helped achieve physical activity and independence-preserving privacy. The Smart homes movement links housing, technology, engineering, sociology, and healthcare in relation to robotics, sensors, telehealth, ergonomics, communications, social care, and safety. Most Smart-home technologies could be used with little assistance or training. Some safety concerns were identified related to malfunctioning of technology; highlighting the importance of contingency systems for events such as power outages

Wireless body area sensor networks (WBANs) can provide specific information about an individual's behavior without using complex laboratory equipment or interfering with one's natural behavior. WBANs are built around several sensing devices wirelessly linked using narrow band radio communication. New wireless communication platforms are based on different protocols and technologies (Wi-Fi, WiMax, Bluetooth, ZigBee, Universal mobile telephone system (UMTS), Ultra wide band (UWB)). These technologies offer a wide range of characteristics in terms of speed, transmission range, power requirements, connectivity, and cost. Accurate recognition of human expressions, emotions, intent, gestures, voice, and body language is being increasingly identified using technology.

1.8 Telehealth and telerehabilitation

On-site technology-enabled, beneficiary friendly contactless telemonitoring is more likely to be accepted by seniors. This will increase independence and enable available healthcare services to improve healthcare outcomes [32]. Telehealth care systems could measure bed and chair occupation and detect falls, taking into account privacy concerns of in-home monitoring systems, older people's attitudes toward assistive telemonitoring systems, and acceptability of video-based home monitoring technologies that capture data about daily activities. Batsis et al. point out that clinicians are required to promote domiciliary telecare for elders [33]. Enforcing compliance and adherence in taking medication is particularly difficult among seniors. Veterans administration (VA) primary care physicians have used video, as a tool to address this [34]. Telerehabilitation is an emerging practice that uses communications technology for the remote delivery of rehabilitative care [35-37]. The Tampa Smart Home was created to assist cognitive rehabilitation in patients with traumatic brain injury. Face recognition was combined with gesture recognition and lip reading [38].

1.9 Internet and Smart homes

According to a recent International telecommunication union (ITU) report, the number of mobile-cellular telephone subscriptions is greater than the global population. More the half the world now use the Internet with 60% of households having internet access [39]. Penetration rates are even more in developing countries. Internet use has become a major defining factor in human progress [40]. While Internet use has increased exponentially over the past two decades, still 27% of older adults aged 65+ in the United States are offline. Only 15% of older adults aged 65+ mostly go online via their Smart phone, the lowest rate of all American adult age groups. Even among older adults who are online, the majority (73%) say they would need help setting up and using new electronic devices. As such, older adults' eHealth literacy, or the ability to access and use health information to make informed healthcare decisions, tends to be low and requires extensive assistance. Further, caregivers of older adults tend to be similarly disadvantaged, particularly those who are nonwhite, of lower education, and without regular healthcare. Social media networks, video chats, and even virtual reality (VR) enable seniors to be more connected, drawing them into mentoring and tutoring programs. Specialized e-career platforms can match retirees with opportunities to utilize their skills [41]. Many older persons have limited access to digital technologies and lack necessary skills to fully exploit them. While half the world's population has Internet access, older persons remain disproportionately offline. In the United

Kingdom, 4.2 million people aged 65 and older have never used the Internet. Older persons in less developed countries are least likely to have access to digital technologies. Visual and hearing impairments, amplify the crisis.

1.10 IoT and Smart homes

Elderly persons with multiple comorbidities often have to be shifted for specialized care. It has been postulated that sensors in large area networks can be affixed on walls. Placing sensors on intelligent carpets or floors could detect a deviation in pattern of walking. Wearables such as a necklace with sensors can unobtrusively monitor vital physiological parameters. Smart objects could intercommunicate and influence physiological state of the individual with mood, sound, and lighting [42]. Embedded sensors can monitor the door passively for unusual events and send an appropriate alert. Smart thermostats can adjust temperature of individual rooms. Electronic hardware and computer software can provide passive monitoring, reminders, entertainment, and information. Advances in sensors and computing help make accurate forecasts about meaningful changes in health, monitoring disease progression, and tracking response to treatments.

With advent of the digital age and plethora of Internet of Things (IoT) there has been a substantial rise in amount of data gathered by these devices in different sectors such as transport, environment, entertainment, sport, and health. By end of 2020, over 2314 exabytes (1 exabyte = 1 billion gigabytes) of data will be generated globally from the health sector. IoT Smart devices alone in the global healthcare market would have a value of US $543.3 billion by 2025 [43]. IoT is an emerging technology connecting everyday devices and systems such as sensors, actuators, appliances, computers, and cellular phones, leading toward a highly distributed intelligent system capable of communicating with other devices and human beings. Smart homes with integrated e-health and assisted living technology is an example of an IoT application that can revolutionize the healthcare system for the elderly. In a Smart home, sensors and actuators are connected through a personal area network or wireless sensor network. Wearable biomedical sensors such as electrocardiogram, electromyogram, electroencephalogram, body temperature and oxygen saturation (SpO_2) sensors can be connected in a wireless body area network (WBAN) or body sensor network to obtain automated, continuous, and real-time measurement of physiological signals [44]. Lack of interoperability among Smart devices, platforms, and systems is a major concern. Motion sensors such as accelerometers, gyroscopes, and magnetometers, in contrast, are smaller, simple to use, and low-power devices suitable for monitoring human activities in a wearable platform. These motion sensors along with vital signs sensors can be embedded in socks, armbands, and t-shirts to receive comprehensive information about the overall health status of the subjects. Smart beds embedded with vital signs sensors are other attractive solutions for monitoring elderly health as well as their sleep quality during sleep.

Built around wireless sensor nodes located throughout a Smart home, some systems require only five sensors, a gateway that supports ZigBee, and links to the internet. Installed in less than an hour using simple QR codes, inexpensive applications do not require any programming, and caregivers or family members can manage it using a smartphone or tablet. The five sensors (motion detection or open/close) are placed in predefined, carefully selected locations to make the system effective: the front door, bedroom, bathroom, refrigerator, and living room. The sensors provide full-home coverage, even through concrete floors and walls. Other RF devices in the house, do not interfere with the sensors [45]. Secure servers store the data analytics, which contain very little personal information. Access is limited to family and caregivers who have been granted permission and users can manage access and permission profiles at any time. With integrated RF filtering, advanced power management, and in-depth design expertise for IoT, communication controllers are available for multiple Smart home sensors and devices, including thermostats, motion sensors, smart plugs, key pads, and door/window sensors. At US $100 for setup and $20–30 per month, it is not very expensive. This makes independent living an accessible choice for increased peace of mind, helping elderly parents, and their children privately share lifestyle information.

1.11 Artificial Intelligence and chatbots in Smart geriatric rehabilitation

With most elders having some health issues, an Artificial intelligence (AI) chatbot companion at home can add value and provide "smarter care" at home in many ways. These include enabling medication reminders, contacting caregiver/children in case of emergencies, encouraging activities, fixing doctors' appointments, and providing reminders. Fear of falling and loneliness are major challenges that most seniors face. Bots need to be programmed to combat loneliness, anxiety, and confusion. AI-enabled robots need to have the emotional intelligence to meet emotional, social, cultural, and physical needs of the elderly. AI today is designed to make purely logical decisions using predictive insights. Adding a blend of emotional, social, cultural, and physical insights to a chatbot would go a long way. Present-day strategy is focused on developing basic AI capabilities in a home companion. Eventually AI integration in elderly care robotics will improve quality of life and independence, monitoring wellness, health, and treatment.

Silver index, is a novel AI-based algorithm to accurately predict and prevent, the risk of falls in the elderly. 30% of those over 65 suffer from falls each year. This is the second leading cause of accidental injury and death worldwide. In Europe, the European Public Health Association estimates that 2.3 million go to the emergency room and 1.5 million are hospitalized. In the United States, older adult falls cost about $50 billion a year. The algorithms analyze 130 biomechanical and clinical parameters providing training suggestions with 200 exercises and 30 protocols, leading to 95% accuracy in predicting falls [46]. Smart Connected Healthcare refers to obvious data-collecting devices such as home glucose and blood pressure monitors and also mobile apps that track and evaluate daily jogs. Temperature detecting sensors in a bra could help detect potential breast cancers. Other monitoring systems for at-risk elderly people living alone will also be available eventually. These data are generally not covered by existing U.S. medical data privacy laws such as HIPAA [47].

Assistive technologies are designed to maintain older peoples' independence and increasing safety. Human–computer interaction technologies include humanoid robots, exoskeletons, rehabilitation robots, service robots, and companion-types.

Psychosocial and ethical issues include intrusive nature of technology solutions. Gerontechnology involves multiple scientific disciplines such as geriatric medicine, psychology, social sciences, computer sciences, engineering and design, informatics, and economics. Cochrane database reviews highlight lack of evidences to support or refute use of SHTs within health and social care [48]. AI has potential to fill gaps in elderly care. Today, there is an immense opportunity to deploy wearable devices that can monitor health and notify emergencies such as falls triggering alerts to distant caregivers. Wearables also aid in ambient monitoring for care facilities acting as social companions, and optimizing care. Medication management systems can help with compliance [49].

1.12 Robots for geriatric rehabilitation

A robot is an autonomous machine capable of sensing its environment, carrying out computations to make decisions, and performing actions in the real world. Many are complicated, from an engineering and a usability point of view. Availability, cost, and effectiveness are all being looked into [50]. Most current robots do not think for themselves. They are driven by remote control or follow hard-coded well-defined paths. If unpredicted conditions occur the robot cannot adapt. Telepresence robots are used to consult with patients and for patients to connect with remote family members. Robot pets have the potential to address loneliness and improve cognition in the elderly. A cuddly seal one of the first therapeutic interactive pets, originally selling for about $5000, is intended for use in elder-care facilities

Sexbots are a delicate subject to discuss. There are many moral and ethical concerns regarding these machines, especially as robots become smarter. Nevertheless, within the rehabilitation patient population, there are many people who have limited abilities and limited opportunities to fulfill their sexual needs. For this group, sexbots have potential to significantly improve quality of life and overall happiness. In the past few years, sexbots have become much more sophisticated. Roxxxy was introduced in 2010 for approximately $5000 and featured a variety of options. Harmony became available in 2017 for approximately $12,000 and has some limited conversational abilities. Humanoid and pet robots, such as NAO and PARO, produce improvements in cognition. Exploding elderly populations of affluent countries are resulting in increasing numbers of age-related cognitive decline. Deep Learning and related technologies are positively impacting robot cognitive training for those experiencing age-related cognitive decline. Human robot interaction with highly patient-centered cognitive training will play an important role [51]. Robots are increasingly being used in neuro-rehabilitation. These devices can assist in practicing upper or lower limb movements and motor relearning, and in developing proprioception, cognitive functions, and attention. The emphasis is on highly repetitive, interactive, and personalized therapy. Most of the devices make it possible to exercise in a virtual environment. It is easier to introduce VR technically than practicing in a real environment. AI in robots should give further options. Robots are not simply supplementary therapists reducing human efforts when executing dull and exhausting exercises [52].

1.13 Deployment of AI and advanced technology in Smart homes

Advantages of machine learning include the ability to handle extremely large numbers of variables in complex environments such as geriatric rehabilitation in Smart homes [53]. Machine learning (ML) is used in symbiotic neuroprosthetics, myoelectric control, and brain computer interface technology. Artificial cognitive applications have been used to judge rehabilitative exercise based on the machine's indications. VR-enabled conventional cognitive rehabilitation enhances motivation for rehabilitation. Memory and attention, in older adults with Minimal Cognitive Impairment, appear to be better with virtual reality based conventional cognitive rehabilitation (VRCCR) [54]. Intelligent mobile and wearable devices collect data, providing users with information to assess health and monitor progress toward individualized rehabilitation goals. Socially and physically assistive robots can be used to help people recuperate after illness or injury, bridging gaps caused by sensory, motor, or cognitive impairments. VR allows individuals to become immersed within and interact with 3D computer-generated simulated environments. Augmented reality (AR) allows computer-generated VR to be superimposed over live "real-world" video imagery. This allows information about the surrounding environment of the user to be available for interaction and digital manipulation to augment the user's perception of the world. VR and AR systems have been used for motor function training and recovery after stroke and in pain management. Mirror therapy, for example, entails the use of a glass mirror to provide visual feedback to the brain. AR mirror systems use a high-resolution video screen and video cameras to simulate a mirror reflection. Thus, the technology allows a person to look into the simulated mirror to see a computer-generated image (e.g., a limb) or other images created by AR. Brain machine interfaces allow the brain to incorporate an artificial neuroprosthetic "tool" into its own cognitive space and use it as an extension of the user's body. "Simple tools" become "intelligent tools" by coadaptation. The tool becomes functionally involved in the extraction and definition of the user's goals. By designing adaptive controls and AI into the neural interface, tools can become active assistants in goal-directed behavior and further enhance human performance particularly for those challenged [55].

1.13.1 Smart toilets

Smart toilets are likely to play an increasingly important role in Smart homes. A Japanese firm Toto created a Smart toilet to monitor health indicators in the early 2000s. Sugar levels in urine, body weight, temperature, and hormone levels were detected. Data were transmitted automatically to computers and doctors. Toto's Flow Sky toilet measured urine flow by monitoring water levels in the toilet. Changes in urine flow could indicate a prostate or bladder problem. A toilet seat developed by Rochester Institute of Technology had sensors to measure blood oxygenation levels, heart rate, and blood pressure [56]. Smart toilets could also help monitor public health. Data from Smart toilets in public spaces could give early warnings of a disease outbreak. Automated analysis of human feces could be beneficial detecting markers of various diseases. An Internet-connected toilet with discreetly placed sensors and AI could analyze breakdown products in urine and feces waste, detecting early signs of disease [57]. Unlike wearable health and fitness trackers, one need not put them on or recharge them. In September 2018, Panasonic released a health-tracking toilet in China that tests the urine for blood and protein. Embedded sensors measured body fat. The Smart toilet is being developed at Stanford University in Palo Alto, CA that [58] can take pictures of the feces, track how often one defecates, and measure how long each defecation takes. AI evaluates consistency of the poop. The toilet also can measure the number of white blood cells and types of protein in urine. Gambhir a Stanford University Professor, passionate about Smart toilets is testing prototypes, which will analyze the user's waste, identifying the person by using fingerprint sensors embedded in the flush handle [59]. The results are sent to the cloud or an app on a Smart phone prompting the user to schedule a doctor appointment. A number of sensors are housed on the underside of the seat, including a camera and a cartridge with paper strips that change color when they come into contact with different substances in the urine, such as blood or sugar. When motion sensors detect a person sitting down, the cartridge slides into view and samples urine on its way into the bowl. As different individuals may use a specific toilet, anal prints can be used to identify the individual. Everyone's anus has unique curves and other patterns. It is distinct, like a fingerprint. As individuals may be squeamish about anal photographs the camera could be replaced with an infra-red or laser scanner. The output here will not resemble a photo. Smart toilets are being used for early detection of irritable bowel syndrome, prostate cancer, or kidney failure in its current stage of development, the toilet can measure 10 different biomarkers [60]. Japan is the world leader in Smart toilets. As 33% of the Japanese population is above the age of 60, self-opening toilet seats, self-cleaning bowls, and a range of toilet accessories exist to aid Japan's aging population [61].

1.13.2 Smart mirrors

Mirrors are an integral part of our daily life. The ability to display information makes a mirror "Smart." Smart mirror technology is now being used to predict and to monitor aspects of health and disease. A combination of intelligent hardware and software could identify subtle, yet clinically relevant changes in physique and appearance. A Smart mirror could record and evaluate body position and motion to identify posture and movement issues, and offer feedback for corrective actions. New challenges in engineering, machine learning, computer vision, and biomedical research need to be addressed The second generation of Smart mirrors fits within a growing set of technologies that integrate monitoring systems with personalized information and computer vision to help individuals achieve their health goals and have a more significant role in healthcare. These devices embed multimodal sensors—multiple cameras, motion detection, lasers, microphones, speakers—as well as software based on AI. This ensures communication with multiple sources of data, linking them to other Smart products and the cloud. This enables noninvasive unobtrusive physiological measurements, creating interactive capabilities based on tracking and recognizing gestures.

Medical Mirrors encourage people to track their vital signals on a daily basis. Computer vision captures an optical signal, reflected off a person's face. Small deviations in reflections can be analyzed and detected. Fit Mirror increases motivation and activity. Movements in front of the mirror result in an interactive display suggesting invigorating physical challenges. Wize Mirror estimates cardio-metabolic risk and anxiety levels from anthropometric measurements of facial features, on the premise that physical characteristics and facial expressions provide surrogate measures. There is of course a danger that this could be yet another illustration of a solution being developed and then going in search of a problem. Cameras embedded in the bathroom mirror or elsewhere in the home could help to more passively predict health issues before they manifest clinically. The technical challenge is to create a mirror camera that can acquire retinal fundus photos automatically without requiring the aid of an additional lens [62]. A Smart mirror can function as Amazon's Alexa or Google's Home Assistant [63].

1.14 Influence of COVID-19 on growth of Smart homes and geriatric rehabilitation

Compliance with increasing regulations and some global restrictions on free travel with extension of partial lockdowns is having a major effect on seniors. The COVID-19 pandemic is inadvertently resulting in a radical transformation in the deployment of technology, particularly in geriatrics. This section reviews the world literature and demonstrates how we are becoming future ready. Smart homes and technology-enabled geriatric rehabilitation will no longer be a question of if but rather a question of when. Older adults are in triple jeopardy during COVID-19: (1) they are more likely to develop serious conditions with higher mortality, (2) less likely to obtain high-quality information or services online, and (3) more likely to experience social isolation and loneliness. Finding financial resources for rapid well-coordinated implementation of digital infrastructure is the biggest challenge. Center for Disease Control and Prevention has advised all elders to "stay home as much as possible." Older adults' adoption and use of technology is less. Older adults should experience "physical distancing" rather than "social distancing" [64]. Shielding older adults from the virus could have adverse side effects. These include increased social isolation, delayed medical treatment, and challenges in meeting basic needs [65].

Due to present physical distancing guidelines, face-to-face neuropsychological assessments necessarily have to be replaced with virtual visits [66]. Supporting older adults with dementia and maintaining their well-being during COVID-19 is of public health concern. Information and communication technology (ICT) may help participation in social networks and communities. Smart phones, tablets, Smart home systems, robots, and VR have also been used in dementia care delivery. Memory and orientation problems support, care delivery, medication management, cognitive interventions, leisure and activities, caregiver education, and support and training need to be addressed. Virtual Cognitive Stimulation Therapy is an example of how technology can be used to deliver group intervention for people with dementia during pandemic-necessitated periods of self-isolation [67]. Mild cognitive impairment is a common condition prevalent among seniors worldwide. With partial lockdowns and restricted transport, deployment of technology is now being looked at as a stand-alone or assisted aid in Smart Homes [68]. Assistive technologies may enable older adults to "age in place," that is, remain living in their homes for longer periods of time. Americans prefer to maintain independent households as long as possible [69].

Rapid adoption and acceptance of technologies at home for quarantine, work, and study due to the pandemic is rescripting the very concept of privacy. Touch biometrics is being replaced with facial recognition entry systems. This could result in access to real-time health records. To stay at home, the government, authorities, employers, landlords need to be let in using digital technologies. The speed with which these technologies are being accepted and adopted is driven by the pandemic as people adjust their lives to lockdown. Rapidity implies thoroughly thinking through their potential impacts. Technology could mean that heightened surveillance and control may persist postpandemic also. Increased digital surveillance would lead to more debate and even resistance [70]. With more people staying at home there will be more adoption of IoT technology. A larger base of IoT users will lead to user upgrades and more new technology development. Ease of installation, integration with other IoT devices, and security will remain key priorities for consumers. Product design must be done with customer experience at the forefront, using Smart monitoring processes to identify and preempt outages or other issues [71].

Integrating Smart home monitoring and collecting personal health data points (temperature, activity, heart rate) alongside environmental data (air quality or occupancy) would help in the wider response and engagement for Smart city health management [72]. Most older adults have limited access and cognizance of Internet and Smart phones. Those familiar with online services might have decline in their physical activity or may be dependent on others. While social media could be a tool to prevent loneliness, boredom, and tediousness in youngsters this is not always true for elders. Mass quarantine and transport restraint has constricted activities of older adults. These include regular walk-and-talk in the park, acquaintance meetings, voluntary service, social care, and congregational gatherings. Contact with plants and animals are reducing, and there is increasing difficulty in accessing prescribed nutrition, medication, and treatment. Social isolation, social distancing, social disconnectedness, and loneliness were found to be mediated with depression and anxiety [73].

The resilience of the elderly can be amazing, if adequately cared for. It has been opined that how one treats seniors during this disaster will shape future treatment [74]. Between one-third and half of older adults across the world and in India have reported varying degrees of loneliness and social isolation prior to the onset of COVID-19 pandemic. Older adults have been most frequently isolated in their residence, cut-off from physical contact with friends and families. Social engagements and community gatherings—the most important source of integration of the older adult in the community—have been suspended. Physical contact—an important component of intimacy and reassurance in old age—has been discouraged.

Virtual interaction through phone calls, video conferencing, and social media have emerged as an alternative form of social engagement. However, the accessibility of Smart devices in older adults is poor, particularly in developing countries (digital exclusion). Adult protective services, day-care centers, community centers, and home visits by health and social workers have been disrupted. Frequent phone and video calls by friends, family members, and caseworkers to check in on the older adult would go a long way toward mitigating isolation and feelings of disconnectedness. Older adults require handholding to make the transition to digital services [75]. Reports from northern Italy suggest that older patients are not getting adequate mental health services as they have limited access to Internet services and Smart phones [76]. Contrary to general perception there are reports suggesting that "Digital screen time" is reduced for the elderly to prevent misinformation and panic. The elderly might have unique requirements in terms of technology handling, communication, and accessibility. This needs to be taken into account while designing digital helplines and teleconsultations [77].

COVID-19 places even more importance on independent living while also ensuring positive mental health and wellbeing. SHT can ensure safety at home and staying connected socially through the Internet. The pandemic has been a catalyst for change accelerating development of future-ready products and services. AI-driven solutions can even be installed remotely. Virtual home care can be deployed through medication management, check-ins, video calling, exercise videos, and more [78]. Radio broadcasts, print notifications, and text messages may make available critical information [79].

Rehabilitation may be necessitated due to movement restrictions, social isolation, and inability to access healthcare for pre-existing or new non-COVID-19 illnesses. Strategies to deliver effective rehabilitation in a COVID-19 world would be different and complex requiring specialist multidisciplinary multiagency services. Deconditioning and frailty as a result of self-isolation, shielding, and social distancing will also require therapy services. Older COVID-19 survivors could have additional cardiorespiratory and neurological deficits. All aspects of rehabilitation and different models of service delivery need to be learnt combining personnel, knowledge, and skills from specific rehabilitation services. Needs based, individualized approach, close to home will enable older people to live well for longer in spite of COVID-19 [80]. Older people, often frail and subject to multiple morbidities are at highest risk for COVID-19. The Association for Geriatric Palliative Medicine rightly promotes the integration of a palliative care approach and skills, into the care of elderly and very elderly people, both in the inpatient setting and at home. Advance care planning is of crucial importance, as most people would prefer to die, not in an intensive care unit, but in their familiar environment [81].

Goodman et al. have reported Television-based telehealth support using TV-Assist Dem, which demonstrated a potential for cognitive stimulation and performing memory exercises as an intellectual activity. TV could also be watched as a recreational activity and to access COVID-19 information, TV-Assist Dem included a digital set-top-box service based on Android technology with a television-based interface, a webcam, and a centralized back-end service with a web-based interface. TV-Assist Dem facilitates remote support through data transmission and video interactivity between users, caregivers, and healthcare professionals [82].

1.15 Smart homes and geriatric rehabilitation: a peep into the future

Rehabilitation is critical when communication between the brain, spinal cord, and peripheral nerves has broken down. Artificial neurons responding to electrical stimuli are now being thought of. Researchers at the University of Bath opine that the synthetic neurons require just 140 nW, or one-billionth the power required by a microprocessor. These synthetic neurons can be used in bioelectronic implants to respond in real time, simulating living neurons [83]. Smart cities have a proliferation of different types of sensors spread across with high bandwidth communication infrastructures, providing unlimited network connectivity. Smart cities infrastructure is being leveraged to provide a Smart healthcare system. In the future, Smart Homes will talk to the Smart city's infrastructure to provide contextualized health-related recommendations and suggestions. This will involve use of computer vision, natural language processing, speech recognition, network planning, machine learning, and data science [84]. Smart Homes presuppose interoperability among the world's leading vendors.

Amazon, Apple, and Google have agreed to create an open-source standard for Internet-connected home products, such as Smart speakers. They will work with Zigbee Alliance, an association of companies working on open IoT standards, plus Samsung, Ikea, and other major players in the sector. The companies have set up a working group, called "Project Connected Home over IP" (or CHIP), which will meet, discuss, and hopefully agree on a set of standards. If adopted by all the major players, this standard could kick start adoption of SHT. An open ecosystem, better security standards, and the rollout of 5G could be a winning combination to push Smart homes into the mainstream [85]. Maintaining mobility is fundamental to independent living and quality of life of older people. Assisted technology in geriatric care and rehabilitation will include use of robots and telehealth. Robotic and sensor technologies could make a significant difference in the lives of older people and their caregivers. Sensors and robotics embedded in the environment (furniture, walls, ceiling, etc.) will offer enhanced support to maintain ADLs. Voice-controlled intelligent personal assistants (e.g., Amazon Echo and Google Home) will be much more interactive and provide companionship, reminders, emergency communication, and even entertainment for older people living alone, thus increasing caregivers' free time [86]. Dynamic Time Warping pattern-matching algorithms applied at run time will be able to compare humanoid with human-operated process sequences. This could reduce time to be spent by human caregivers. A robot could appear before the senior, gain his/her attention, and speak inviting to follow physical exercises showing the correct sequence of movements. Personalized rehabilitation programs could be offered [87].

The "new aged" will have more purchasing power and higher levels of familiarity with technology. Expectations will be higher. Being more fit, active, mobile, safe, connected, independent, and self-reliant with an excellent quality of life will be the new mantra. Avoiding "getting old" would even be regarded as an option. Geography independent, access to cost-effective mobile broadband services will be deemed a constitutional right. A rapidly emerging "Smart homes" movement could occur worldwide. Establishing the validity, efficacy, practicality, and cost of Smart homes technologies and proof that it does indeed make a difference will be required [88].

1.16 Conclusions

Success in deployment of technology for clinical rehabilitation purposes hinges on understanding who will use it and how it will help them to achieve their goals. It is the patient's goals that matter and technology is just another tool we use together to help achieve them. What really matters is helping others win—even if it means slowing down and changing our course now and then. As a septuagenarian belonging to the BC (Before Computers not Before COVID-19!) era the author though a technology buff is able to understand the necessity for getting into the minds of the end user, "Customer delight" is not just a cliché used as marketing ploy. The solution should not go in search of a problem, we need to develop what is required never forgetting that the world has turned upside down and that the present-day octogenarians have come from another planet!

Acknowledgments

The secretarial assistance of Ms Lakshmi is acknowledged.

References

[1] Reshaping the future of senior living in the post pandemic world. https://www.hindustantimes.com/health/covid-19-reshaping-the-future-of-senior-living-in-the-post-pandemic-world/story-WXUU3fvqMpKhgfLDE8hg6I.html.
[2] Why social distancing is a big worry for senior citizens. https://economictimes.indiatimes.com/news/politics-and-nation/covid-19-why-social-distancing-is-a-big-worry-for-senior-citizens/printarticle/74866566.cms.
[3] To be a senior citizen during India's COVID-19 epidemic. https://science.thewire.in/health/to-be-a-senior-citizen-during-indias-covid-19-epidemic/.
[4] W. Miller Thomas, Smart advances in healthcare for geriatric patients, Am. J. Biomed. Sci. Res 1 (3) (2019).
[5] M.E. Morris, B. Adair, K. Miller, E. Ozanne, R. Hampson, et al., Smart-home technologies to assist older people to live well at home, Aging Sci 1 (2013) 101.
[6] Adela Sitar, Dan Sitar, Oana Cramariuc, Vasile Negrean, Dorel Sampelean, Rusu Lucia, Olga Orasan, Adriana Fodor, Gabriela Dogaru, Angela Cozma, Smart homes for older people involved in rehabilitation activities - reality or dream, acceptance or rejection?, Balneo Res. J 9 (2018) 291–298.
[7] The new frontier for artificial intelligence: senior care. https://www.winimy.ai/blog/the-new-frontier-for-artificial-intelligence-senior-care/.
[8] M. Birks, M. Bodak, J. Barlas, J. Harwood, M. Pether, Robotic seals as therapeutic tools in an aged care facility: a qualitative study, J. Aging Res 2016 (2016) 8569602 10.1155/2016/8569602.
[9] I. Dutzi, M. Schwenk, M. Kirchner, et al., What would you like to achieve?" goal-setting in patients with dementia in geriatric rehabilitation, BMC Geriatr. 19 (2019) 280. https://doi.org/10.1186/s12877-019-1296-7.
[10] M.A. McCaskey, A. Schättin, A.L. Martin-Niedecken, E.D. de Bruin, Making more of IT: enabling intensive motor cognitive rehabilitation exercises in geriatrics using information technology solutions, BioMed. Res. Int. 2018 (2018) 4856146. https://doi.org/10.1155/2018/4856146.
[11] J.F. Bean, A.R. Orkaby, J.A. Driver, Geriatric rehabilitation should not be an oxymoron: a path forward, Arch. Phys. Med. Rehabil 100 (5) (2019) 995–1000.
[12] Geriatric rehabilitation. https://emedicine.medscape.com/article/318521-overview.
[13] M.U. Hassan, Nadia Mumtaz, AI in assisting the elderly and people with disabilities, Int. J. Res. Eng 3 (2016) 35–39.
[14] L. Liu, E. Stroulia, I. Nikolaidis, A. Miguel-Cruz, A. Rios Rincon, Smart homes and home health monitoring technologies for older adults: a systematic review, Int. J. Med. Inform 91 (2016) 44–59.
[15] Ghazal Bilal, Khatib Khaled, Smart home automation system for elderly, and handicapped people using XBee, Int. J. Smart Home 9 (2015) 203–210.
[16] M.E. Jacob, P. Ni, J. Driver, E. Leritz, S.G. Leveille, A.M. Jette, J.F. Bean, Burden and patterns of multimorbidity: impact on disablement in older adults, Am. J. Phys. Med. Rehabil 99 (5) (2020) 359–365.
[17] L.N. Lee, M.J. Kim, A critical review of Smart residential environments for older adults with a focus on pleasurable experience, Front. Psychol 10 (2020) 3080.
[18] George Demiris, Brian Hensel, Smart Homes" for patients at the end of life, J. Hous. Elderly 23 (1-2) (2009) 106–115.

[19] L.E. van Dokkum, T. Ward, I. Laffont, Brain computer interfaces for neurorehabilitation—its current status as a rehabilitation strategy post-stroke, Ann. Phys. Rehabil. Med. 58 (2015) 3–8.

[20] M.I. Cajita, N.A. Hodgson, K.W. Lam, S. Yoo, H.R. Han, Facilitators of and barriers to mHealth adoption in older adults with heart failure, Comput. Inform. Nurs 36 (8) (2018) 376–382.

[21] S.J. Parker, S. Jessel, J.E. Richardson, M.C. Reid, Older adults are mobile too! Identifying the barriers and facilitators to older adults' use of mHealth for pain management, BMC Geriatr 13 (2013) 43.

[22] A. Spann, E. Stewart, Barriers and facilitators of older people's mHealth usage: a qualitative review of older people's views, Hum. Technol. 14 (2018) 264–296.

[23] M. V. Foster, K. A. Sethares, Facilitators and barriers to the adoption of telehealth in older adults, Comput. Inform., Nurs. 32 (2014) 523–533.

[24] J. Coughlin, L.A. D'Ambrosio, B. Reimer, M.R. Pratt, Older adult perceptions of smart home technologies: implications for research, policy & market innovations in healthcare, Proc. Annual International Conference of the IEEE Engineering in Medicine and Biology Society, 2007 1810–1815.

[25] S.T. Peek, K.G. Luijkx, M.D. Rijnaard, M.E. Nieboer, C.S. van der Voort, S. Aarts, J. van Hoof, H.J. Vrijhoef, E.J. Wouters, Older adults' reasons for using technology while aging in place, Gerontology 62 (2) (2016) 226–237.

[26] K.L. Courtney, Privacy and senior willingness to adopt Smart home information technology in residential care facilities, Methods Inf. Med 47 (1) (2008) 76–81.

[27] D. Pal, S. Funilkul, N. Charoenkitkarn, P. Kanthamanon, Internet-of-Things and smart homes for elderly healthcare: an end user perspective, IEEE. Access 6 (2018) 10483–10496.

[28] Technology acceptance model. Wikipedia. https://en.wikipedia.org/wiki/Technology_acceptance_model#:~:text=The%20technology%20acceptance%20model%20(TAM,people%20to%20use%20the%20technology.

[29] WWW '17 Companion: In: Proc. 26th International Conference on World Wide Web Companion. 2017 Pages 1095–1101. https://doi.org/10.1145/3041021.3054928.

[30] Smart homes for the elderly. https://www.smarthome.com/blogs/tips-tricks/smart-homes-for-the-elderly.

[31] For the elderly, smart homes mean the promise of more freedom. https://www.networkworld.com/article/3073519/for-the-elderly-smart-homes-mean-the-promise-of-more-freedom.html.

[32] A.H. Sapci, H.A. Sapci, Innovative assisted living tools, remote monitoring technologies, artificial intelligence-driven solutions, and robotic systems for aging societies: systematic review, JMIR Aging 2 (2) (2019) e15429 doi: 10.2196/15429.

[33] J.A. Batsis, P.R. DiMilia, L.M. Seo, K.L. Fortuna, M.A. Kennedy, H.B. Blunt, P.J. Bagley, J. Brooks, E. Brooks, S.Y. Kim, R.K. Masutani, M.L. Bruce, S.J. Bartels, Effectiveness of ambulatory telemedicine care in older adults: a systematic review, J. Am. Geriatr. Soc 67 (8) (2019) 1737–1749.

[34] W. Chang, M. Homer, M.I. Rossi, Use of clinical video telehealth as a tool for optimizing medications for rural older veterans with dementia, Geriatrics. (Basel) 3 (3) (2018) 44 30.

[35] N. Tyagi, R. Aikat, Tele-rehabilitation as an adjunct service for geri care: reaching the unreached, Int. J Sci. Res 4 (2015) 19–21.

[36] B. Roxanna, H. Kathleen, L. Charles, Using telerehabilitation to support elders with chronic illness in their homes, Topics Geriatr. Rehabil 23 (2007) 47–51.

[37] H. Mathieu, F. Rejean, B. Patrick, In-home telerehabilitation for geriatric patients, IEEE Eng. Med. Biol. Mag. 27 (2008) 29–37.

[38] D.T. Barry, Adaptation, artificial intelligence, and physical medicine and rehabilitation, PM&R 10 (2018) S131–S143.

[39] New ITU statistics show more the half the world is now using the Internet. https://news.itu.int/itu-statistics-leaving-no-one-offline/.

[40] Smartphone ownership and internet usage continues to Climb in emerging economies. https://www.pewresearch.org/wp-content/uploads/sites/2/2016/02/pew_research_center_global_technology_report_final_february_22__2016.pdf.

[41] Smart cities: digital solutions for a more livable future. McKinsey Global Institute. 2018. https://www.mckinsey.com/industries/capital-projects-and-infrastructure/our-insights/smart-cities-digital-solutions-for-a-more-livable-future#.

[42] G. Edelmayer, Paul Panek, Peter Mayer, Wolfgang Zagler, Technologies for Smart toilets., Mstnews: Bimonthly Journal for Micro and Nano Technologies 05 (14-16) (2005) 35.

[43] Z. Allam, D.S. Jones, On the coronavirus (COVID-19) outbreak and the smart city network: universal data sharing standards coupled with artificial intelligence (AI) to benefit urban health monitoring and management, Healthcare. (Basel) 8 (1) (2020) 46.

[44] S. Majumder, E. Aghayi, M. Noferesti, H. Memarzadeh-Tehran, T. Mondal, Z. Pang, M.J. Deen, Smart homes for elderly healthcare-recent advances and research challenges, Sensors. (Basel) 17 (11) (2017) 2496.

[45] Smart Homes for seniors: how the IoT can help aging parents live at home longer. https://www.qorvo.com/design-hub/blog/smart-homes-for-seniors-how-iot-helps-aging-parents.

[46] Novel AI based algorithm for falls prediction for adults over 65 years. https://www.prnewswire.com/news-releases/novel-ai-based-algorithm-for-falls-prediction-for-adults-over-65-years-301125029.html.

[47] Smart Home, smart health, smart cars: what will inter-connected devices mean for users and data users? https://www.insightsassociation.org/article/smart-home-smart-health-smart-cars-what-will-inter-connected-devices-mean-users-and-data.

[48] A. Pilotto, R. Boi, J. Petermans, Technology in geriatrics, age and ageing, 47 (6) (November) (2018) 771–774. https://doi.org/10.1093/ageing/afy026.

[49] M. L. Noone, Artificial Intelligence in Geriatrics—Geriatrics & Gerontology Initiative: International. Workshop on care of the elderly, BMH Med. Journal 7(Suppl) (2020). (Ahead of Print). https://www.babymhospital.org/BMH_MJ/index.php/BMHMJ/article/view/231/528.

[50] D.D. Luxton, L.D. Riek, Artificial intelligence and robotics in rehabilitation, in: L.A. Brenner, S.A. Reid-Arndt, T.R. Elliott, R.G. Frank, B. Caplan (Eds.), Handbook of Rehabilitation Psychology, American Psychological Association, Washington DC, 2019, pp. 507–520. https://doi.org/10.1037/0000129-031.

[51] A.A. Vogan, F. Alnajjar, M. Gochoo, Khalid S. Robots, AI and cognitive training in an era of mass age-related cognitive decline: a systematic review, IEEE Access 8 (2020) 18284–18304.

[52] G. Fazekas, I. Tavaszi, The future role of robots in neuro-rehabilitation, Expert Rev. Neurother. 19 (2019) 471–473.

[53] D. Anderson, Artificial intelligence and applications in PM&R, Am. J. Phys. Med. Rehabil. 98 (2019) e128–e129.

[54] J.-S. Park, Y.-J. Jung, G. Lee, Virtual reality-based cognitive–motor rehabilitation in older adults with mild cognitive impairment: a randomized controlled study on motivation and cognitive function, Healthcare 8 (2020) 335.

[55] J.C. Sanchez, B. Mahmoudi, J. DiGiovanna, et al., Exploiting co-adaptation for the design of symbiotic neuroprosthetic assistants, Neural Netw. 22 (2009) 305–315.

[56] Artificial intelligence in your toilet. yes, really! https://www.forbes.com/sites/bernardmarr/2019/05/20/artificially-intelligent-toilets-yes-they-are-here/?sh=67bb0b07626d.

[57] Here's how smart toilets of the future could protect your health https://www.nbcnews.com/mach/science/here-s-how-smart-toilets-future-could-protect-your-health-ncna961656.

[58] Waiting for a 'smart' toilet? It's nearly here. https://www.sciencenewsforstudents.org/article/smart-toilets-are-almost-here.
[59] 'Smart toilet' recognizes users and checks for signs of disease. https://www.medicalnewstoday.com/articles/smart-toilet-recognizes-users-and-checks-for-signs-of-disease.
[60] 'Smart toilet' monitors for signs of disease. https://med.stanford.edu/news/all-news/2020/04/smart-toilet-monitors-for-signs-of-disease.html.
[61] Smart toilets make more sense than most Smarthome Tech. https://www.reviewgeek.com/23196/why-would-anyone-want-a-smart-toilet/.
[62] R. Miotto, M. Danieletto, J.R. Scelza, et al., Reflecting health: Smart mirrors for personalized medicine, NPJ Digital Med. 1 (2018) 62. https://doi.org/10.1038/s41746-018-0068-7.
[63] What is a smart mirror - smart mirror guide. https://smartmirrorguide.com/what-is-a-smart-mirror/.
[64] Bo Xie, Neil Charness, Karen Fingerman, Jeffrey Kaye, Miyong T. Kim, Anjum Khurshid, When going digital becomes a necessity: ensuring older adults' needs for information, services, and social inclusion during COVID-19, J. Aging Social Policy 32 (4-5) (2020) 460–470.
[65] E. A. Miller, Protecting and improving the lives of older adults in the COVID-19 era, J. Aging Social Policy 32 (4-5) (2020) 297–309.
[66] D. E. Marra, K. M. Hamlet, M.Bauer Russell, Dawn Bowers, Validity of teleneuropsychology for older adults in response to COVID-19: a systematic and critical review, Clin. Neuropsychol. 34 (7-8) (2020) 1411–1452, doi:10.1080/13854046.2020.1769192.
[67] G. Cheung, K. Peri, Challenges to dementia care during COVID-19: innovations in remote delivery of group cognitive stimulation therapy, Aging Ment. Health (2020), doi:10.1080/13607863.2020.1789945.
[68] N.A. Basarudin, A.L. Yeon, Z.M. Yusoff, N.H.M. Dahlan, N. Mahdzir, Smart home assisted living for elderly: the needs for regulations, J. Social Sci. Res. 6 (2018) 7–13.
[69] M.E. Pollack, Intelligent technology for an aging population: the use of AI to assist elders with cognitive impairment, AI Mag 26 (2005) 9–24.
[70] Maalsen S., Dowling R. Covid-19 and the accelerating smart home. Big Data & society. 2020. doi: 10.1177/2053951720938073.
[71] COVID-19 impact on the Smart home experience. http://www.parksassociates.com/blog/article/covid-19-impact-on-the-smart-home-experience-insights-from-sutherland.
[72] COVID-19 a boon for smart home? https://www.broadbandtechreport.com/in-the-home/article/14173205/covid19-a-boon-for-smart-home.
[73] S. Mukhtar, Psychological impact of COVID-19 on older adults, Curr. Med. Res. Pract 10 (4) (2020) 201–202.
[74] D. Banerjee, M.M. D'Cruz, T.S. Sathyanarayana Rao, Coronavirus disease 2019 and the elderly: focus on psychosocial well-being, agism, and abuse prevention—An advocacy review, J. Geriatr. Ment. Health 7 (2020) 4–10.
[75] M. D'cruz, D. Banerjee, An invisible human rights crisis': the marginalization of older adults during the COVID-19 pandemic—An advocacy review, Psychiatry. Res 292 (2020) 113369.
[76] G. Serafini, E. Bondi, C. Locatelli, M. Amore, Aged patients with mental disorders in the COVID-19 era: the experience of Northern Italy, Am. J. Geriatr. Psychiatry 28 (7) (2020) 794–795.
[77] D. Banerjee, Age and ageism in COVID-19': Elderly mental health-care vulnerabilities and needs, Asian J. Psychiatr. 51 (2020) 102154. doi: 10.1016/j.ajp.2020.102154.
[78] Guest article: the importance of smart home technology and collaboration in the 'next normal'.http://attoday.co.uk/guest-article-the-importance-of-smart-home-technology-and-collaboration-in-the-next-normal/.

[79] The Impact of COVID-19 on older persons. United Nations Report. https://unsdg.un.org/sites/default/files/2020-05/Policy-Brief-The-Impact-of-COVID-19-on-Older-Persons.pdf.
[80] S. De Biase, L. Cook, D. A. Skelton, M. Witham, R. ten Hove, The COVID-19 rehabilitation pandemic, Age Ageing 49 (5) (2020) 696–700. https://doi.org/10.1093/ageing/afaa118.
[81] R. Kunz, M. Minder, COVID-19 pandemic: palliative care for elderly and frail patients at home and in residential and nursing homes, Swiss Med. Wkly 150 (2020) w20235.
[82] J.M. Goodman-Casanova, E. Dura-Perez, J. Guzman-Parra, A. Cuesta-Vargas, F. Mayoral-Cleries, Telehealth home support during COVID-19 confinement for community-dwelling older adults with mild cognitive impairment or mild dementia: survey study, J. Med. Internet. Res 22 (5) (2020) e19434.
[83] AI goes out on a limb for rehabilitation. https://eandt.theiet.org/content/articles/2020/04/ai-goes-out-on-a-limb-for-rehabilitation/.
[84] SmartCare: futuristic health care system for smart cities. Heba Aly, Tongyang Li, Richard Neal, Manaswi Saha, Rashmi Sankepally. Department of Computer Science, University of Maryland. 2015. https://wiki.cs.umd.edu/cmsc798F_s16/images/6/6b/Summary_B8.pdf.
[85] Amazon, Apple and Google joining forces could be what makes smart homes happen. MIT technology review. 2019. https://www.technologyreview.com/2019/12/19/131479/amazon-apple-and-google-joining-forces-could-be-what-makes-smart-homes-happen/.
[86] E.B. Mukaetova-Ladinska, T. Harwood, J. Maltby, Artificial Intelligence in the healthcare of older people, Arch. Psychiatr. Ment. Health 4 (2020) 7–13.
[87] M. Simonov, G. Delconte, Humanoid assessing rehabilitative exercises, Methods Inf. Med. 54 (2015) 114–121.
[88] Smart technologies for older people. http://farseeingresearch.eu/wp-content/uploads/2012/07/MORRIS-Smart-technologies-for-older-people-MEG2.pdf.

CHAPTER

2

Smart home technology for geriatric rehabilitation and the Internet of Things

Riitta Mieronkoski[a], *Iman Azimi*[b], *Lydia Sequeira*[c], *Laura-Maria Peltonen*[d]

[a]Department of Nursing Science, University of Turku, Turku, Finland, [b]Department of Computing, University of Turku, Turku, Finland, [c]Institute of Health Policy, Management & Evaluation, University of Toronto, Toronto, ON, Canada; Centre for Addiction and Mental Health, Toronto, ON, Canada, [d]Department of Nursing Science, University of Turku, Turku, Finland

LEARNING OBJECTIVES

After reading this chapter you will be able to:

- Describe contemporary Internet of Things-based systems available for geriatric rehabilitation
- Understand a geriatric rehabilitation service user as Internet of Things user
- Assess the potential and challenges with the use of Internet of Things-based systems in geriatric rehabilitation

2.1 Introduction

The Internet of Things (IoT) consists of multiple technologies embedded with sensors and software to gather and exchange information with systems over the Internet. Traditional perspectives on the use of the IoT are connected with Smart homes [1-2], but these technologies also show

Smart Home Technologies and Services for Geriatric Rehabilitation
DOI: https://doi.org/10.1016/B978-0-32-385173-2.00006-0

great potential in geriatric rehabilitation with individuals suffering from chronic conditions such as Parkinson, cardiac conditions [3], stroke [3-4], and fall-related injuries [3]. Complex health issues, which are caused by chronic comorbidities and geriatric syndromes, pose challenges to the effective and timely rehabilitation of older adults.

The IoT-based systems offer new means to measure and monitor health conditions for both formative and summative evaluation of geriatric rehabilitation and health outcomes. It enables real-time and smooth data exchange between professionals to support care provision. However, many issues warrant attention for the safe and efficient development and implementation of the IoT-based systems in geriatric rehabilitation. These regard the quality of the technology used, risk of infection from malware, privacy and confidentiality issues [5-7] as well as a lack of user competence [8-9]. This chapter focuses on the potential, measured benefits and challenges with the use of the IoT-based systems from a transdisciplinary health professionals' perspective.

2.2 The IoT and the rehabilitation process

Rehabilitation is an interactive process between a patient and health professionals, which aims to maintain or restore the best possible function in various areas of life. In geriatric rehabilitation, the focus lies on "*restoring functional ability or enhancing residual functional capability in older people with disabling impairments*" [10].

The rehabilitation process is based on a systematic plan and patient-centered objectives. In geriatric rehabilitation, these are set by involving the older adult, the family members, as well as the multiprofessional team members of health professionals. The rehabilitation process can be described through the following phases: the assessment phase, which includes the examination and clinical reasoning for the diagnosis; the rehabilitation phase, which covers selected interventions targeted to restore or enhance functional ability; and the evaluation phase, which targets the assessment of the outcomes achieved. A recent review [3] suggests that the IoT-based systems could be applied in all of these phases. These systems could support the functional diagnoses in the evaluation phase, help to monitor the exercises or activities during the intervention phase, and support in measuring the outcomes in the final evaluation.

The use of IoT-based systems in rehabilitation may help to maintain the contact between the service user and the health professionals in various settings by enabling continuous data flow of monitored features of movement, such as activity levels, intensity of the exercises, and specific features of the movements. These systems can include wearable sensors and instrumented rehabilitation devices that are connected to smartphones or tablets. The health professionals can monitor the quality and quantity of the interventions in real-time and increase compliance via personalized goal setting and instructions [11]. Moreover, the goal of meaningful participation has lately been emphasized in geriatric rehabilitation in addition to mobility and self-care activities [12]. The IoT-based systems could be used for strengthening the role of the older adult as an active participant in the rehabilitation process and in involving the informal caregivers in the rehabilitation process.

2.3 Technical perspectives on the IoT

The IoT is a network of Smart objects that collect data, interconnect with each other, and communicate with remote servers over the Internet [13,14]. Such a network exploits a distinct set of paradigms—such as communication infrastructures, shared pools of data, and artificial intelligence—to provide high quality and effective services. The use of the IoT-based systems is dramatically increasing particularly in healthcare devices and well-being applications due to the advances in embedded systems, wireless communication, and data analytics. At-risk population groups (e.g., the older adults) can be ubiquitously monitored, leveraging the IoT-based systems that are enabled by Smart energy-efficient lightweight wearable devices [15].

IoT-based systems can be conventionally partitioned into three main layers: the sensor network, the gateway, and the cloud server. A view of such a system is shown in Fig. 2.1. The sensor network consists of Smart devices, which acquire data from the entities and their environment. For example, smartwatches and Smart rings—enabled by photoplethysmography sensors and accelerometers—are used to track various vital signs at home, in clinics, and in hospitals. In this layer, smartphones can also collect data from the user's physical activity and location. In addition, other sensors can be exploited to acquire environmental parameters (e.g., ambient light) that enable situation-aware applications. Such devices are equipped with communication modules (e.g., Bluetooth and Wi-Fi), by which the data are shared with the other nodes. The gateway acts as a communication bridge between the sensor network and the cloud server. The gateway layer, including multiple fixed or mobile devices, is located in the vicinity of the sensor network. It allows lightweight local data analytic services and data transmission over the Internet [16]. Third, the cloud server is responsible for data storage, data analysis, and security and privacy management. The cloud layer tailors the shared knowledge collected from the sensors and data analytic techniques (e.g., machine learning) to provide accurate and individualized decision support. The cloud server provides the data, models, and results for health professionals, or family members and caregivers, depending on the context. It can also send notifications to the end-users in case of an emergency.

IoT-based systems are exploited to collect a large amount of data throughout the health monitoring process. Advanced data analytic

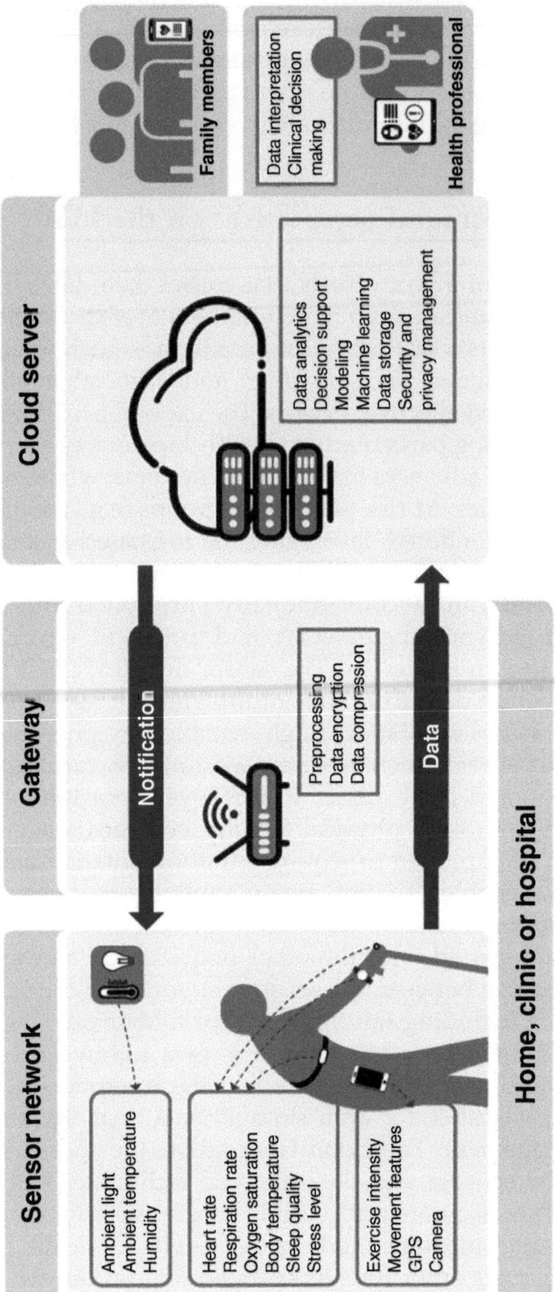

FIG. 2.1 The Internet of Things–based system in geriatric rehabilitation.

approaches are required in this regard to fuse the collected data and extract new information and knowledge. The data are acquired from diverse sources (e.g., sensors) in different conditions. Therefore, a preprocessing step—including noise reduction and data filtering—is needed to improve the data quality. Such processing is necessary for biosignals, such as photoplethysmogram, as motion artifacts affect the signal's and vital signs' quality. Moreover, artificial intelligence and machine learning algorithms are required for detection, prediction, and prevention applications. Such algorithms can leverage user's data to train models, enabling health deterioration detection and personalized decision-making [15,16].

The data analytic approaches can be performed in the gateway devices and cloud servers (see Fig. 2.1). On the one hand, gateway devices can employ lightweight approaches to enable various services such as early detection and local notification with minimum latency [16]. The gateway devices are bounded by limited computational capacity; however, their services do not rely on degraded access to Internet connections during monitoring. On the other hand, cloud servers, equipped with powerful computational resources, can implement machine learning algorithms—including deep learning—that is enabled by health history data [17,18]. Such algorithms are used to satisfy various system-driven and data-driven attributes such as accuracy, reliability, resiliency, and energy efficiency [18,19].

2.4 Security and privacy and the IoT

Data security and privacy play an important role in the IoT-based systems and in particular in health monitoring applications targeted to vulnerable groups, such as older adults. The security and privacy issues need to be acknowledged on all three main layers of the IoT-based systems [20-22]. The sensor network includes various nodes (e.g., physical devices) that are small and operate in dynamic environments. The sensor network is susceptible to different threats, as attackers might physically access the devices [20-21]. The locally stored data in the devices should be encrypted and access should be limited. Moreover, the sensor nodes interconnect with each other via wireless technologies (e.g., WiFi). In this regard, an entity might be untrusted, or the collected data may need to be shared with some specific devices. Therefore, authentication methods should be employed and secure connections are required.

The gateway devices act as a bridge between the sensor network and remote servers. These devices are susceptible to data breaches, so authentication and privacy-preserving schemes are essential [23-24]. Unauthorized access and eavesdropping in this layer cause critical security problems for data confidentiality and privacy. For example, personal data might be at risk of privacy breaches when a communication channel fails if the key exchange method is not secure. Security mechanisms such as encryption should be employed in this regard. Moreover, intrusion detection methods can be exploited to track the traffic and behavior of the nodes.

The cloud servers also require security mechanisms to manage data privacy, authenticity, integrity, and confidentiality [25]. The cloud servers store the collected data and share the data with other entities. Thus, reliable and secure communication channels should be ensured. For example, access control, authentication, authorization, and data encryption methods are necessary. The security issues might even be magnified in the cloud servers due to Big Data with high volume, velocity, and variety [26].

2.5 The development process of IoT-based systems

Developing an IoT-based system for specific areas in healthcare, such as geriatric rehabilitation, demands transdisciplinary cooperation between several stakeholders, including specialists from engineering, information technology, computer science, healthcare, and enterprises. The starting point of any technological solution targeted at the healthcare setting should be the identification of the end-users needs [27], that is, the geriatric rehabilitation service users and health professionals, the therapists, and the rehabilitation physicians.

The development of IoT-based systems involves hardware and software development of several layers as well as usability testing in clinical environments. Defined by the WHO, systems used for diagnosis, monitoring, or medical intervention, which aim to treat, relive symptoms, or compensate for injury, should be approved as medical devices. Regulation on the development and use of such devices differs regionally. For example, in Europe, the development of medical devices is regulated by the European Union Medical Device Regulation [28] and in the United States of America the development process is controlled by the Food and Drug Administration regulations [29]. According to the medical device development process, the initial preclinical phase focuses on the ideation and needs assessment, including the user's requirements as well as the literature reviews to explore contemporary knowledge on the topic. In the next phase, the prototype is developed and tested for feasibility in an iterative process. The validity of the device is assessed and the premarket evaluation is conducted, where after the final regulatory decisions, product launch and post-market monitoring follow [30].

2.6 Competency needs of developers and users

The development of IoT-based systems for geriatric rehabilitation requires competence in the rehabilitation process, the specific needs and resources associated with the older adults, as well as the technologies embedded with sensors and software that gather and exchange information with systems over the Internet. Hence, a transdisciplinary approach is needed for successful development outcomes. From the developers' perspective, understanding the users' unique needs and requirements is vital. However, the role of end-users in the development process of these systems is still underutilized. Medical device users are most often only involved in the development process during the usability testing [31]. However, the usability testing is complex in itself and defined through five dimensions, including learnability, efficiency, memorability, error resistance and remediation, and satisfaction [32]. However, there are some examples of development studies involving older adults to evaluate the usability of IoT-based technologies. For example, one study [33] involved older adults with mild dementia, including memory impairment and decline in cognitive abilities, to evaluate passive positioning alarms.

From the health professionals' perspective, their workflow can be greatly modified with the use of IoT-based systems to support more integrated and personalized patient care within geriatric rehabilitation. This leads often to a shift in required competencies. New competencies required relate to being able to broaden the technological literacy across both software and hardware domains. This will maximize the use of these new technologies and the teaching and supporting of patient self-care, which includes supporting how a patient uses the technology or interprets the data produced, also acknowledging the data privacy and security aspects [34]. Barakat and colleagues [35] have discussed competencies across several domains, including:

- knowledge base regarding technologies (e.g., how to collect health-related data or what to do if the technology does not work),
- attitudes toward technology (e.g., conveying empathy through videoconferencing),
- analytical skills (e.g., how to interpret data collected to support clinical decision-making),
- general guiding skills (e.g., ability to assess the needs and preferences of the patient with respect to the technology),
- communication skills (e.g., ability to interpret nonverbal and verbal expressions during remote monitoring), and
- an understanding of privacy and confidentiality issues (e.g., understand regulations and how to minimize risk of data breaches).

In terms of older adult end-users, barriers to adoption of IoT-based systems (i.e., tablet computers) may include a lack of instructions and guidance, a lack of knowledge and confidence, as well as feelings of inadequacy [36]. Thus, competencies for this group of end-users include overcoming these barriers and being able to understand instructions or being able to find or ask for additional education when required. Other barriers include age-related changes, such as vision and hearing loss and fine motor difficulties [37], which correlate with physical competencies required to make full use of technologies within geriatric rehabilitation.

2.7 IoT-based systems and implications for geriatric rehabilitation

IoT-based systems offer promising solutions for objective and continuous monitoring of health indicators to support clinical decision-making and reduce caregiver burden. These systems allow monitoring health using wearable devices such as wristbands, smartwatches, smart textiles, belt-worn PCs, and Smart glasses [38]. Although the literature reviews synthesizing research on IoT-based systems in geriatric rehabilitation are scarce, reviews from the perspective of older adults in general have identified several ways how these systems can support care of older adults. These include monitoring of aged care and chronic conditions, activity recognition, clinical applications, emergency conditions, mental health, movement disorders, rehabilitation, prevention, providing accessibility to care providers and service users [39], as well as daily life monitoring and independent living [40], and falls prevention and detection [40,41]. Also, reviews on the literature on the IoT-based systems developed for broader populations provide an insight into technologies that may be helpful in geriatric rehabilitation, such as systems developed for gait analysis [42,43] and upper-limb rehabilitation [44].

A conventional review describes a number of subtopics in geriatric rehabilitation including frailty, comprehensive geriatric assessment, admission screening, assessment tools, interdisciplinary teams, hip fracture, stroke, nutrition, dementia, and depression [45,46]. A variety of examples of IoT-based systems align with these topics. For example, systems for remote monitoring after hip fracture [47], gait detection for stroke patients [48], location tracking for patients with dementia [49], wearable cameras for improving depressive symptoms and memory of patients with Alzheimer's disease [50], and systems to improve nutritional knowledge and skills of older adults [51]. Samples of IoT-based systems with possible implications for geriatric rehabilitation are presented in Table 2.1 with a description of the technology used, suggested support for geriatric rehabilitation, and results of the evaluation of the presented system.

2.8 User perspectives on the IoT

Over 70% of those aged 65 years and over use the Internet and 59% have broadband. A large majority of these users (71%) use the Internet regularly, despite the unique challenges facing the older adults in terms of

TABLE 2.1 Examples of Internet of Things–based systems with implications for geriatric rehabilitation.

Purpose of technology	Description of technology	Potential support for geriatric rehabilitation	Evaluation results
Remote health monitoring [52]	Data on heart rate, temperature, and blood oxygenation levels of older adults are collected through a wearable Internet of Things–based system (i.e., biometric bracelet) and communicated in real time to mobile applications of professionals and family members.	May provide information of vital signs to professionals and family for care planning.	Evaluation was done with five healthy adults using the System Usability Scale. The usability was interpreted as very good.
Remote monitoring in rehabilitation of older adults after hip fracture [53]	The system consists of two sensor systems, a wearable activity monitor and a sensor monitoring system in the home of the older adult. The wearable activity monitor is worn on the hip. It measures daily activities.	May provide professionals with information about daily activities for rehabilitation after hip fracture.	Feasibility testing with older adults showed that the system was easy to use.
Remote health monitoring and fall detection [54]	The system consists of a wearable sensing device, a gateway, and a cloud. It measures the electro cardio gram (ECG) as well as kinematic data for the identification of arrhythmias. Also ECG biometric recognition and fall detection are integrated. Collected information can be transmitted to the professional.	May provide information for early intervention as well as trends of cardiac rhythm for care planning.	The evaluation of the system was focused on energy consumption of the sensors.
Remote health monitoring and fall detection [55]	An IoT-based system for older adults that collects real-time information from in-home sensors. The system can detect falls and alert professionals and family members in occurrence of unexpected changes in routines.	May provide information about temperatures and falls for care planning.	Technical testing showed good performance regarding system functionalities.

(continued)

TABLE 2.1 (Cont'd)

Purpose of technology	Description of technology	Potential support for geriatric rehabilitation	Evaluation results
Fall detection [56]	A motion detection system, which is built on passive radio frequency identification labels for the monitoring of the status of older adults.	May provide information about sudden falls for early intervention with older adults.	Experiment in students' dormitory showed that the system distinguished a fall from other actions.
Fall detection [57]	A motion detection system based on a three-axis accelerometer, gyroscope. and magnetometer, in addition to a barometer sensor estimates the posture and altitude of the older adult.	May provide information about the movement and sudden falls for early intervention with older adults and trends for care planning.	Evaluation reached 100% of sensitivity in testing protocols with volunteers who performed different types of falls. The combination of these sensors and used algorithms led to better performance when compared to other similar systems.
Remote bladder monitoring [58]	An implantable wireless and battery-less bladder pressure monitoring system for use in lower urinary tract dysfunction. This system monitors the real-time bladder situation by an implanted sensor that transmits signals to an external receiver with Bluetooth low energy.	May provide information to implantable nerve stimulators on bladder pressure with older adults with neurogenic bladder for improving therapies with neurostimulator devices as well as outcomes.	In-vitro system validation and in-vivo experiment on animals showed that the implant seems suitable for long-term battery-free operation in vivo.
A home-based frailty detection system [59]	A wireless automatic home-based frailty detection system is based on four devices. First, the eScale simulates the traditional falling ruler for measuring reaction time. Second, the eChair measures pressure exertion through a pressure sensor. Third, the ePad detects footsteps and can be used for balance tests. Fourth, the eReach measures displacement through ultrasound sensors.	May provide information for the monitoring of the impact of aging among older adults for care planning.	The system was tested with frailty measures, including reaction time, balance, functional reach, physical weakness, and slowness of movement (n=8). The proposed system correlated with traditional tests.

Gait analysis in stroke rehabilitation [48]	A gait analysis system that consists of a built-in sensor in the smartphone and a shoe, which is connected to the Internet. The system monitors insole pressure and accelerations of motion to identify abnormal gait patterns. Real-time monitored data can be sent to a professional and family member.	May provide information about walking patterns for the prediction of cautious gait and warn about abnormal gait to prevent fall.	Based on testing with participants (n=10), the system was able to identify and predict cautious gait, which may lead to falls.
A web-based system for monitoring of motion of older adults with Parkinson's disease [60]	A system that contains a data collection engine based on wearable sensors, web services, and a graphical user interface, which has a video conferencing option. The data can be used to estimate clinical scores, which indicate severity of bradykinesia, dyskinesia, and tremor.	May provide information about patients with Parkinson's' disease to support the care planning and titration of medications.	Technical testing indicated that the system may be suitable for use in the monitoring of motion of older adults with Parkinson's disease.
A mobile system for home-based monitoring of Parkinson's disease [61]	A mobile cloud-based mHealth app that collects information about Parkinson's disease, including hand tremor and waking motion through a smartphone 3D accelerometer. The system builds on computing performance and cloud service storage for analyzing progression and severity of the disease.	May provide information for the monitoring and evaluation of motor function in Parkinson's disease.	Evaluations showed that the system caught motion features to separate tremor and reductions in the severity of gait.

technology use, such as physical challenges, skeptical attitudes, or difficulties learning new technologies [62]. Specific user data for those older adults undergoing rehabilitation are unavailable. The IoT-based systems enable users to share their rehabilitation progression on the Internet not only with professionals, but also with family, friends, and peers; however, there is not a clear consensus for data ownership, data privacy, and data sharing regarding these systems [63], which may cause additional concern across the healthcare context.

It is necessary to understand user perspectives of the IoT-based applications to consider the usability and deployment challenges of monitoring applications from an all-inclusive top view [64]. Many studies have reported that user-acceptance remains to be a large challenge, including hardware and software ease-of-use, comfortability, weight, size, and energy consumption [38]. The acceptance of the technology by the elderly after implementation is influenced by a vast variety of issues, which can be categorized into six domains, including concerns regarding the appropriate function of the technology, user-friendliness, expected benefits, experienced need for use, social influence, and characteristics of the user [65].

Previous research on end-user perspectives on the IoT-based systems has shown in a survey of older adults across Asia that user adoption could be largely explained by the effort expectancy, which refers to "the degree of ease associated with the use of any system" [66]. Hence, it is important to involve older adults within the codesign and governance of Smart health technologies and Smart homes, as end-user advice, perceived trust and perceived cost of the application are factors associated with older adults' acceptance of technology, but unfortunately, these views are frequently ignored [67].

2.9 Evidence of the effectiveness of IoT-based systems

There has been a drastic increase in the research literature on IoT-based systems targeted at the health setting during the last five years. However, only scarce research on the use of these systems can be found on implications specifically for geriatric rehabilitation. Most research focuses on these technologies on elderly in general or on other medical areas such as neurology, cardiology, psychiatry, or psychology [68]. A majority of IoT-based systems developed for the geriatric setting concern monitoring and supporting elderly people to have an independent lifestyle including safety aspects, while other areas, such as the prevention of pressure ulcers, have received far less attention [39]. Further, only 14% of studies on the use of sensors in the health setting were related to rehabilitation based on a current review [69]. The interchangeable use of IoT-related terms in the literature reflects a rapidly emerging area of research and indicates a need for concept analysis [68].

Some evidence exists to support the use of IoT-based technologies to reduce falls [70]; however there is in general limited evidence on technology readiness for digital technologies supporting ageing in place after system implementation, as only a minority of research published has studied mature technologies [65,68]. Furthermore, a gap in the literature exists on research explaining how technology supports aging in place with randomized controlled trials in genuine situations, as well as on research exploring the long-term effectiveness of these technologies [71]. Research has also shown challenges with the use of these technologies regarding size and usability of the device, accuracy and reliability of collected data, poor feature extraction due to artifacts, data loss, data privacy and safety issues, data processing issues, and low user acceptability [40]. However, individual studies have shown an opportunity for improvements in care with IoT-based systems. Examples include improved accuracy in monitoring of Parkinson's disease symptoms with the use of wearable devices [72], and improved daily functioning among older adults recovering from hip fracture, when using sensor monitoring–informed occupational therapy instead of care as usual [73].

2.10 Current state and future vision of the use of IoT in geriatric rehabilitation

The literature on the IoT-based systems specifically focusing on geriatric rehabilitation is scarce; however, there are a vast number of these technologies which have been developed for rehabilitation elsewhere and for supporting older adults in general. Although these systems can be used for several different purposes and conditions and may be difficult to categorize [69], many of these systems have implications for geriatric rehabilitation. The evidence on the effectiveness of IoT-based systems in geriatric rehabilitation is scarce; nonetheless, these technologies show great potential in the field. The majority of current IoT-based systems seem to be in an early stage of maturity. The objectives of these systems focus on issues such as fall detection, health monitoring, gait assessment, or conditions such as Parkinson and dementia. User groups of these technologies include health professionals, but also the older adults themselves and their family members. In the future, these technologies may support better engagement of older adults and family members in the rehabilitation process, by empowering them to take more active roles within their own care as decision makers and goal setters.

Health professionals need sufficient competence in understanding the implications, possible benefits, and risks with the development and adoption of IoT-based technologies in geriatric rehabilitation. Structures to support in-service education and transdisciplinary collaboration, as well as clearly defined responsibilities in using these technologies, are necessary for appropriate development, safe adoption, and effective use. The development and implementation work needs a strong involvement of end-users to ensure appropriateness and usability. Additionally, issues regarding data security, confidentiality, validity, and reliability of the technologies used need to be acknowledged. Ethical implementation requires systematic planning and monitoring of use. In the future, these technologies could have a major role when ensuring effective and equally accessible rehabilitation to the older adults.

References

[1] M.Z. Uddin, W. Khaksar, J. Torresen, Ambient sensors for elderly care and independent living: a survey, Sensors. (Basel) 18 (7) (2018) 2027, doi:10.3390/s18072027.

[2] S. Arlati, V. Colombo, D. Spoladore, L. Greci, E. Pedroli, S. Serino, P. Cipresso, K. Goulene, M. Stramba-Badiale, G. Riva, A. Gaggioli, G. Fserrigno, M. Sacco, A social virtual reality-based application for the physical and cognitive training of the elderly at home, Sensors. (Basel) 19 (2) (2019) 261, doi:10.3390/s19020261.

[3] Câmara Gradim L. C., Archanjo José M., Marinho Cezar da Cruz D. and de Deus Lopes R., Internet of Things services and applications in rehabilitation: an interdisciplinary and meta-analysis review IEEE Trans. Neural Syst. Rehabil. Eng., 28, 9, 2043-2052, 2020, doi: 10.1109/TNSRE.2020.3005616.

[4] D. Schließmann, M. Nisser, C. Schuld, T. Gladow, S. Derlien, L. Heutehaus, N. Weidner, U. Smolenski, R. Rupp, Trainer in a pocket - proof-of-concept of mobile, real-time, foot kinematics feedback for gait pattern normalization in individuals after stroke, incomplete spinal cord injury and elderly patients, J. Neuroeng. Rehabil 15 (1) (2018) 44, doi:10.1186/s12984-018-0389-4.

[5] A. Subahi, G. Theodorakopoulos, Detecting Internet of Things user behavior and sensitive information in encrypted internet of things-app traffic, Sensors. (Basel) 19 (21) (2019) 4777, doi:10.3390/s19214777.

[6] A. Panarello, N. Tapas, G. Merlino, F. Longo, A. Puliafito, Blockchain and Internet of Things integration: a systematic survey, Sensors. (Basel) 18 (8) (2018) 2575, doi:10.3390/s18082575.

[7] A. Giaretta, N. Dragoni, F. Massacci, Internet of Things security configurability with security-by-contract, Sensors. (Basel) 19 (19) (2019) 4121, doi:10.3390/s19194121.

[8] P.S. de Boer, A.J. van Deursen, T.J. Van Rompay, Accepting the Internet-of-Things in our homes: the role of user skills., Telemat. Inform 36 (2019) 147–156.

[9] A.J. van Deursen, K. Mossberger, Any Thing for Anyone? A New Digital Divide in Internet-of-Things Skills, Policy Internet 10 (2) (2018) 122–140.

[10] Boston working group on improving health care outcomes through geriatric rehabilitation Med Care, 35 (1997), JS4-JS20.

[11] B.H. Dobkin, A rehabilitation-Internet-of-Things in the home to augment motor skills and exercise training, Neurorehabil. Neural Repair 31 (3) (2017) 217–227, doi:10.1177/1545968316680490.

[12] W.P. Achterberg, I.D. Cameron, J.M. Bauer, J.M. Schols, Geriatric rehabilitation—state of the art and future priorities, J. Am. Med. Dir. Assoc. 20 (4) (2019) 396–398.

[13] L. Atzori, A. Iera, G. Morabito, The Internet of Things: a survey, Comput. Netw. 54 (15) (2010) 2787–2805.

[14] A. Al-Fuqaha, M. Guizani, M. Mohammadi, M. Aledhari, M. Ayyash, Internet of Things: a survey on enabling technologies, protocols, and applications, IEEE. Commun. Surv. Tutor. 17 (4) (2015) 2347–2376.

[15] R. Mieronkoski, I. Azimi, A.M. Rahmani, R. Aantaa, V. Terävä, P. Liljeberg, S. Salanterä, The Internet of Things for basic nursing care—a scoping review, Int. J. Nurs. Stud. 69 (2017) 78–90.

[16] A.M. Rahmani, T.N. Gia, B. Negash, A. Anzanpour, I. Azimi, M. Jiang, P. Liljeberg, Exploiting smart e-Health gateways at the edge of healthcare Internet-of-Things: a fog computing approach, Futur. Gener. Comput. Syst. 78 (2018) 641–658.

[17] L.M. Dang, M. Piran, D. Han, K. Min, H. Moon, A survey on Internet of Things and cloud computing for healthcare, Electronics 8 (7) (2019) 768.

[18] I. Azimi, O. Oti, S. Labbaf, H. Niela-Vilen, A. Axelin, N. Dutt, P. Liljeberg, A.M. Rahmani, Personalized maternal sleep quality assessment: an objective IoT-based longitudinal study, IEEE Access 7 (2019) 93433–93447.

[19] A. Anzanpour, D. Amiri, I. Azimi, M. Levorato, N. Dutt, P. Liljeberg, A.M. Rahmani, Edge-assisted control for healthcare Internet of Things: a case study on PPG-based early warning Score, ACM Trans. Internet of Things 2 (1) (2020) 1–21.

[20] X. Chen, K. Makki, K. Yen, N. Pissinou, Sensor network security: a survey, IEEE Commun. Surv. Tutor. 11 (2) (2009) 52–73.

[21] R. Mahmoud, T. Yousuf, F. Aloul, I. Zualkernan, Internet of Things (Internet of Things) security: current status, challenges and prospective measures, In: Proc. 10th International Conference for Internet Technology and Secured Transactions (ICITST), IEEE, 2015, pp. 336–341.

[22] Q. Gou, L. Yan, Y. Liu, Y. Li, Construction and strategies in Internet of Things security system, In: Proc. IEEE International Conference on Green Computing and Communications and IEEE Internet of Things and IEEE Cyber, Physical and Social Computing, IEEE, 2013, pp. 1129–1132.

[23] S. Yi, Z. Qin, Q. Li, Security and privacy issues of fog computing: a survey, Proc. International Conference on Wireless Algorithms, Systems, and Applications, Cham, Springer, 2015, pp. 685–695.

[24] M. Mukherjee, R. Matam, L. Shu, L. Maglaras, M.A. Ferrag, N. Choudhury, V. Kumar, Security and privacy in fog computing: challenges, IEEE Access 5 (2017) 19293–19304.

[25] S. Sicari, A. Rizzardi, L.A. Grieco, A. Coen-Porisini, Security, privacy and trust in Internet of Things: the road ahead, Comput. Netw. 76 (2015) 146–164.

[26] I.A.T. Hashem, I. Yaqoob, N.B. Anuar, S. Mokhtar, A. Gani, S.U. Khan, The rise of "big data" on cloud computing: review and open research issues, Inform. Syst. 47 (2015) 98–115.

[27] M. Ghazali, N.A. Mat Ariffin, R. Omar, User centered design practices in healthcare: a systematic review, In: Proc. 3rd International Conference on User Science and Engineering (i-USEr), ShahAlam, 2014, pp. 91–96, doi:10.1109/IUSER.2014.7002683.

[28] European Parlament. (2017). Regulation (EU) 2017/745 of the European Parliament and of the Council of 5 April 2017 on medical devices. https://eur-lex.europa.eu/eli/reg/2017/745/oj.

[29] Food and Drug Administration (2020) overview of device regulation. https://www.fda.gov/medical-devices/device-advice-comprehensive-regulatory-assistance/overview-device-regulation. (Accessed November 1, 2020).

[30] Center for Devices and Radiological Health & U.S. Food and Drug Administration. 2011. The CDRH Innovation initiative. https://www.fda.gov/about-fda/cdrh-innovation/medical-device-innovation-initiative-white-paper (Accessed 31 January 2021).

[31] H.-M. Matinolli, R. Mieronkoski, S. Salanterä, Health and medical device development for fundamental care: scoping review, J. Clin. Nurs 29 (2020) 1822–1831 https://doi-org.ezproxy.utu.fi/10.1111/jocn.15060.

[32] R.J. Branaghan, Human factors in medical device design: methods, principles, and guidelines, Crit. Care Nurs. Clin. North Am 30 (2) (2018) 225–236, doi:10.1016/j.cnc.2018.02.005.
[33] A. Olsson, K. Skovdahl, M. Engström, Using diffusion of innovation theory to describe perceptions of a passive positioning alarm among persons with mild dementia: a repeated interview study, BMC. Geriatr. 16 (2016), doi:10.1186/s12877-016-0183-8 Article No. 3.
[34] K. Saranto, C. Ronquillo, O. Velez, Nursing competencies for multiple modalities of connected health technologies, Stud. Health Technol. Inform. 232 (2017) 172–182.
[35] A. Barakat, R.D. Woolrych, A. Sixsmith, W.D. Kearns, H.S. Kort, eHealth technology competencies for health professionals working in home care to support older adults to age in place: outcomes of a two-day collaborative workshop, Medicine 2.0 2 (2) (2013) e10.
[36] E. Vaportzis, M. Giatsi Clausen, A.J. Gow, Older adults perceptions of technology and barriers to interacting with tablet computers: a focus group study, Front. Psychol. 8 (2017) 1687.
[37] L. Gitlow, Technology use by older adults and barriers to using technology, Phys. Occup. Ther. Geriatr. 32 (3) (2014) 271–280.
[38] T.G. Stavropoulos, A. Papastergiou, L. Mpaltadoros, S. Nikolopoulos, I. Kompatsiaris, Internet of Things wearable sensors and devices in elderly care: a literature review, Sensors 20 (10) (2020) 2826.
[39] S.Y.Y. Tun, S. Madanian, F. Mirza, Internet of Things (IoT) applications for elderly care: a reflective review, Aging Clin. Exp. Res. 33 (4) (2021) 855–867. doi: 10.1007/s40520-020-01545-9. Epub 2020 Apr 10. PMID: 32277435.
[40] M.M. Baig, S. Afifi, H. GholamHosseini, F. Mirza, A systematic review of wearable sensors and Internet of Things-based monitoring applications for older adults–a focus on ageing population and independent living, J. Med. Syst. 43 (8) (2019) 233.
[41] H. Nguyen, F. Mirza, M.A. Naeem, M.M. Baig, Falls management framework for supporting an independent lifestyle for older adults: a systematic review, Aging Clin. Exp. Res 30 (11) (2018) 1275–1286, doi:10.1007/s40520-018-1026-6. Epub 2018 Sep 8. PMID: 30196346.
[42] C. Wang, X. Wang, Z. Long, J. Yuan, Y. Qian, J. Li, Estimation of temporal gait parameters using a wearable microphone-sensor-based system, Sensors. (Basel) 16 (12) (2016) 2167, doi:10.3390/s16122167.
[43] S. Gill, N. Seth, E. Scheme, A multi-sensor cane can detect changes in gait caused by simulated gait abnormalities and walking terrains, Sensors (Basel), 20, 2020 631, doi:10.3390/s20030631.
[44] L.F. Lin, Y.J. Lin, Z.H. Lin, L.Y. Chuang, W.C. Hsu, Y.H. Lin, Feasibility and efficacy of wearable devices for upper limb rehabilitation in patients with chronic stroke: a randomized controlled pilot study, Eur. J. Phys. Rehabil. Med 54 (3) (2018) 388–396, doi:10.23736/S1973-9087.17.04691-3.
[45] J.L. Wells, J.A. Seabrook, P. Stolee, M.J. Borrie, F. Knoefel, State of the art in geriatric rehabilitation. Part I: review of frailty and comprehensive geriatric assessment, Arch. Phys. Med. Rehabil. 84 (6) (2003) 890–897.
[46] J.L. Wells, J.A. Seabrook, P. Stolee, M.J. Borrie, F. Knoefel, State of the art in geriatric rehabilitation. Part II: clinical challenges, Arch. Phys. Med. Rehabil. 84 (6) (2003) 898–903.
[47] A. Haleem, M. Javaid, I.H. Khan, Internet of Things (Internet of Things) applications in orthopaedics, J. Clin. Orthop. Trauma 11 (2020) S105–S106.
[48] A.J.A. Majumder, Y. ElSaadany, M. ElSaadany, D.R. Ucci, F. Rahman, A wireless Internet of Things system towards gait detection in stroke patients, Proc. IEEE International Conference on Pervasive Computing and Communications Workshops (PerCom Workshops), IEEE, 2017, pp. 449–454.

[49] P.P. Ray, D. Dash, D. De, A systematic review and implementation of Internet of Things-based pervasive sensor-enabled tracking system for dementia patients, J. Med. Syst. 43 (9) (2019) 287.
[50] A.R. Silva, M.S. Pinho, L. Macedo, C. Moulin, S. Caldeira, H. Firmino, It is not only memory: effects of sensecam on improving well-being in patients with mild Alzheimer disease, Int. Psychogeriatr 29 (5) (2017) 741–754, doi:10.1017/S104161021600243X.
[51] F. Lattanzio, A.M. Abbatecola, R. Bevilacqua, C. Chiatti, A. Corsonello, L. Rossi, S. Bustacchini, R. Bernabei, Advanced technology care innovation for older people in Italy: necessity and opportunity to promote health and wellbeing, J. Am. Med. Dir. Assoc 15 (7) (2014) 457–466, doi:10.1016/j.jamda.2014.04.003.
[52] L.A. Durán-Vega, P.C. Santana-Mancilla, R. Buenrostro-Mariscal, J. Contreras-Castillo, L.E. Anido-Rifón, M.A. García-Ruiz, O.A. Montesinos-López, F. Estrada-González, An IoT system for remote health monitoring in elderly adults through a wearable device and mobile application., Geriatrics (Basel) 4 (2) (2019) 34, doi:10.3390/geriatrics4020034.
[53] M.C. Pol, G. Ter Riet, M. van Hartingsveldt, B. Kröse, S.E. de Rooij, B.M. Buurman, Effectiveness of sensor monitoring in an occupational therapy rehabilitation program for older individuals after hip fracture, the SO-HIP trial: study protocol of a three-arm stepped wedge cluster randomized trial, BMC Health Serv. Res 17 (1) (2017) 3, doi:10.1186/s12913-016-1934-0.
[54] I. Boukhennoufa, A. Amira, F. Bensaali, S. Soheilian Esfahani, A novel gateway-based solution for remote elderly monitoring, J. Biomed. Inform 109 (2020) 103521, doi:10.1016/j.jbi.2020.103521.
[55] S. Pinto, J. Cabral, T. Gomes, We-care: an IoT-based health care system for elderly people, In: Proc. IEEE International Conference on Industrial Technology (ICIT), IEEE, 2017, pp. 1378–1383.
[56] L. Zhu, R. Wang, Z. Wang, H. Yang, TagCare: using RFIDs to monitor the status of the elderly living alone, IEEE Access 5 (2017) 11364–11373.
[57] P. Pierleoni, A. Belli, L. Maurizi, L. Palma, L. Pernini, M. Paniccia, S. Valenti, A wearable fall detector for elderly people based on AHRS and barometric sensor, IEEE sensors J 16 (17) (2016) 6733–6744.
[58] Y. Zhong, B. Qian, Y. Zhu, Z. Ren, J. Deng, J. Liu, Q. Bai, X. Zhang, Development of an implantable wireless and batteryless bladder pressure monitor system for lower urinary tract dysfunction, IEEE J. Transl. Eng. Health Med 8 (2019) 2500107, doi:10.1109/JTEHM.2019.2943170.
[59] C.C. Lin, C.C. Chen, P.S. Lin, R.G. Lee, J.S. Huang, T.H. Tsai, Y.C. Chang, Development of home-based frailty detection device using wireless sensor networks, J. Med. Biol. Eng. 36 (2) (2016) 168–177.
[60] B.R. Chen, S. Patel, T. Buckley, R. Rednic, D.J. McClure, L. Shih, D. Tarsy, M. Welsh, P. Bonato, A web-based system for home monitoring of patients with Parkinson's disease using wearable sensors, IEEE Trans. Biomed. Eng 58 (3) (2011) 831–836, doi:10.1109/TBME.2010.2090044.
[61] D. Pan, R. Dhall, A. Lieberman, D.B. Petitti, A mobile cloud-based Parkinson's disease assessment system for home-based monitoring, JMIR Mhealth Uhealth 3 (1) (2015) e29, doi:10.2196/mhealth.3956 Mar 26.
[62] PEW Research Centre. Internet/broadband fact sheet. internet & technology. https://www.pewresearch.org/internet/fact-sheet/internet-broadband/ (Accessed 31 January 2021).
[63] C.F. Pasluosta, H. Gassner, J. Winkler, J. Klucken, B.M. Eskofier, An emerging era in the management of Parkinson's disease: wearable technologies and the Internet of Things, IEEE J. Biomed. Health Inform 19 (6) (2015) 1873–1881, doi:10.1109/JBHI.2015.2461555.

[64] I. Azimi, A.M. Rahmani, Tenhunen H. Liljeberg, Internet of Things for remote elderly monitoring: a study from user-centered perspective, J. Ambient Intelli Humaniz. Comput. 8 (2) (2017) 273–289.

[65] A. Tsertsidis, E. Kolkowska, K. Hedström, Factors influencing seniors' acceptance of technology for ageing in place in the post-implementation stage: a literature review, Int. J. Med. Inform 129 (2019) 324–333, doi:10.1016/j.ijmedinf.2019.06.027.

[66] D. Pal, S. Funilkul, N. Charoenkitkarn, P. Kanthamanon, Internet-of-Things and smart homes for elderly healthcare: an end user perspective, IEEE Access 6 (2018) 10483–10496, doi:10.1109/ACCESS.2018.2808472.

[67] N.H. Chadborn, K. Blair, H. Creswick, N. Hughes, L. Dowthwaite, O. Adenekan, E. Pérez Vallejos, Citizens' juries: when older adults deliberate on the benefits and risks of smart health and smart homes, Healthcare (Basel) 7 (2) (2019) 54.

[68] F. Sadoughi, A. Behmanesh, N. Sayfouri, Internet of things in medicine: a systematic mapping study, J. Biomed. Inform 103 (2020) 103383, doi:10.1016/j.jbi.2020.103383.

[69] L.M.S.D. Nascimento, L.V. Bonfati, M.B. Freitas, J.J.A. Mendes Junior, H.V. Siqueira, SL Stevan Jr, Sensors and systems for physical rehabilitation and health monitoring-A review., Sensors (Basel) 20 (15) (2020) 4063, doi:10.3390/s20154063.

[70] P. Khosravi, A.H. Ghapanchi, Investigating the effectiveness of technologies applied to assist seniors: a systematic literature review, Int. J. Med. Inform 85 (1) (2016) 17–26, doi:10.1016/j.ijmedinf.2015.05.014.

[71] A. Ollevier, G. Aguiar, M. Palomino, I.S. Simpelaere, How can technology support ageing in place in healthy older adults? A systematic review, Public Health Rev 41 (1) (2020) 26, doi:10.1186/s40985-020-00143-4.

[72] M.K. Erb, D.R. Karlin, B.K. Ho, K.C. Thomas, F. Parisi, G.P. Vergara-Diaz, J.F. Daneault, P.W. Wacnik, H. Zhang, T. Kangarloo, C. Demanuele, C.R. Brooks, C.N. Detheridge, N. Shaafi Kabiri, J.S. Bhangu, P. Bonato, mHealth and wearable technology should replace motor diaries to track motor fluctuations in Parkinson's disease, NPJ Digit. Med 3 (2020) 6, doi:10.1038/s41746-019-0214-x.

[73] M.C. Pol, G. Ter Riet, M. van Hartingsveldt, B. Kröse, B.M. Buurman, Effectiveness of sensor monitoring in a rehabilitation programme for older patients after hip fracture: a three-arm stepped wedge randomised trial, Age Ageing 48 (5) (2019) 650–657.

CHAPTER

3

Ageing population supported by ambient-assisted living in the Kingdom of Saudi Arabia

Majid H. Alsulami[a]*, *Anthony S. Atkins*[b], *Ali S. Sorour*[b], *Russell J. Campion*[b]

[a]Department of Computer Science, Community College, Shaqra University, Shaqra, Saudi Arabia, [b]School of Digital, Technologies and Art, Staffordshire University, Stoke-on-Trent, United Kingdom

LEARNING OBJECTIVES

After reading this chapter, you should be able to:

- What are the challenges associated with Geriatric Rehabilitation (GR) and the provision of technology for Ambient Assisted Living (AAL) to support elderly people to live independently, comfortably, and healthily?
- What are the issues associated with an increasing elderly population in the Kingdom of Saudi Arabia in terms of healthcare provision and welfare support for independent living?
- How will an Ambient Assisted Living Home Proactive Monitoring System (AALHPMS) support stakeholders in adopting Smart sensors technology to assist Geriatric Rehabilitation in the Kingdom of Saudi Arabia.
- How will a website (AgeinginKSA.org) support elderly people in social interaction and virtual communities in Geriatric Rehabilitation in the Kingdom of Saudi Arabia.

3.1 Geriatric rehabilitation and ambient-assisted living

Geriatric rehabilitation (GR) is defined as an *"evaluative, diagnostic, and therapeutic interventions whose purpose is to restore functional ability or enhance*

*Community College, Shaqra, Shaqra University, Saudi Arabia.

Smart Home Technologies and Services for Geriatric Rehabilitation
DOI: https://doi.org/10.1016/B978-0-323-85173-2.00005-9

residual functional capability in older adults with disabling impairments" [1]. While GR refers to the medical expression of a set of activities intended to provide better life for elderly people, ambient-assisted living (AAL) technology is defined as *"the provision of sustainable care for the growing number of elderly in their homes or selected living environments, personalized care based on their profile and surrounding context, which will allow them to extend their independent existence"* [2]. AAL, as a technological field, investigates innovations in technology that aids healthcare and rehabilitation for impaired seniors, especially for people with cognitive impairments and who live on their own. These innovations assist them to live independently, comfortably, and healthy [3]. Chorchado et al. [4] provided an intelligent environment called Geriatric Ambient Intelligence (GerAmi) that integrates multiagent systems and different technologies to facilitate the management of geriatric residences [3]. Therefore, AAL is considered to be a technological innovation that is intended to improve the life quality of the elderly and has the capability to support their requirements in their later years through the application of technology [5]. It is developed through automation of homes, and through assistive domesticity. It provides people in this age group (elderly) with assistance in carrying out their daily activities, prolonging their life expectancy, and improving their social life and communication [6].

The number of elderly people in the world is expected to be 1.4 billion by 2030 and 2.1 billion by 2050 and might increase to 3.2 billion by 2100. The growth in the ageing population is rapidly increasing, and their care cost will be a challenging issue in the future [7]. The population of the Kingdom of Saudi Arabia (KSA) in 2015 was 31.5 million and is estimated to be 39.1 million in 2030. This number will increase to 46.1 million in 2050 and reach 47.6 million in 2100. While the Saudi Arabian population continues to increase, the ageing population will also continue to increase rapidly [8].The current status of elderly people in Saudi Arabia (≥60 years) according to the retirement policy in the KSA [9] is controllable, because the proportion is only 5%. However, the ageing population in the KSA will be unmanageable in the future, as the percentage will increase sharply to reach 20.9% in 2050, and will further rise to 33.5% by 2100 [7, 10, 11] . A study conducted in 2013 in the KSA, with 10,735 participants over 60 years of age, showed that 45.8% take medication [12].

A survey of 2095 participants demonstrated the high percentage of risk of obstructive sleep apnea among the elderly (≥60 years), which was 41% [13]. Worldwide, falls are also another major concern among elderly people [14].Heart failure and cardiovascular diseases are considered major concerns that affect elderly people in the KSA [15, 16]. "Cardiac failure is an inability of the heart to deliver blood (and therefore oxygen) at a rate commensurate with the requirements of the metabolizing tissues at rest or during light exercise" [17]. Many elderly people face decline in their health when they become older, and need some form of support in their daily activities, as well as facilities to monitor their health [6, 14, 18].The increase in the ageing population worldwide compared to the increase in the world population presents challenges for both healthcare providers and elderly people [14]. In particular in the KSA, the growing number of people included in the ageing population presents many challenges to the Saudi Arabian Government: (1) the increment of persons requesting pension benefits will increase, (2) the economy will decrease, (3) healthcare expenditures will increase, and (4) spending will be more and saving will be less [10].

These challenges and issues require novel approaches for dependable self-adapting technological innovations. AAL is advocated as a potential form of technology that can provide support in assisting and helping elderly people to overcome their challenges, and to fulfill and meet their needs and requirements as their lives and circumstances change with age. The continuous growth in the number of elderly Saudi Arabians will need a proactive monitoring system (PMS) to assist in maintaining their quality of life, independent living, the chances of living longer, health, and the ability to stay active. The chapter outlines the application of a website referred to as Ageing in the KSA (AgeinginKSA) and is based on prototype system architecture that uses both home-operated static sensors positioned on walls, doors, floors, ceilings, and furniture and wearable technologies such as the Smart medically approved watch for monitoring heart beats and providing a Home PMS (AALHPMS) [19].

3.1.1 AAL technologies

Many technologies and projects have been designed and deployed as Smart environments that can assist elderly people to live independently [20]. Recent AAL advancements include Smart homes, assistive robotics, wearable and mobile devices, [21–23] and e-textiles [21].The origin of Smart home technology dates back to 1970s' home automation technologies [24]. A Smart home can be defined as a *"residence equipped with a high-tech network, linking sensors and domestic devices, appliances, and features that can be remotely monitored, accessed, or controlled, and provide services that respond to the needs of its inhabitants"* [25]. The concept of the Smart home is to allow facilities to provide home care for elderly people in an encouraging and cost-effective manner [26, 27]. Smart homes can be placed into different categories, depending on the equipment and systems installed. The main benefits of Smart homes are: improving healthcare, security and safety, saving energy, ensuring comfort [28], monitoring health conditions, providing remote control and surveillance [29], controlling appliances and devices such as heating and lighting [30], and assisting in performing daily activities [31]. For example, an assisted living Smart home provides elderly people with the help necessary to be independent; it can take action when unusual activities happen, such as contacting a nominated carer [25]. Many technologies and projects have been deployed and tested, such as the LOBIN project, which maintains the location and remotely measures the respiratory rate of elderly people in medical environments [32]. GatorTech Smart House locates its occupants and manages the environment, assessing their mobility in an attempt to improve lifestyle [33]. HOME project uses infrared and biosensors to deliver information to healthcare specialists about elderly people living in the house [34]. A study conducted by Gfk [35] for over 7000 consumers across 7 countries, the Unites States, Brazil, China, United Kingdom, South Korea, Japan, and Germany, reported that 91% of consumers were aware of Smart homes. In addition, the global market share of Smart homes has grown to from US $40 billion to US $58 billion by 2020. The study stated that security and control count for 55% of the consumers' needs, and the major barrier that limits their adoption is cost, for 36% of the study responses. A study indicated that many investigations did not indicate the cost of technologies for a Smart home. However, the same study indicated that two studies it had investigated stated the cost was low. In addition, the same study mentioned that there is a study that said the cost was less than US $400, while another stated that the maximum cost of retrofitting a home was €13,500 [36].

The factors influencing adopting AAL technologies and the use of medically approved Smart watches to monitor heart rates in elderly people have been discussed previously by Alsulami and Atkins [37, 38], and Alsulami et al. [19, 111]. The intention of the system is to provide a proactive and integrated Smart home and AAL sensors, which can provide exception alerts. For example, if an incident occurs (such as loss of heartbeat), the care provider or next of kin can be notified via an SMS message or email and after trying initially to check by phone with the elderly person being monitored for any "false" notification the emergency response protocols would be activated. This would involve notifying designated next of kin/appropriate key holders (these can be amended by the elderly person) and screen sharing on to their Smart in real time to support the elderly person. The knowledge-based system (KBS) would operate via a web portal referred to AgeinginKSA.

3.2 Ageing population

According to the United Nations, the world population in 2019 was 7.71 billion. This number is projected to reach 8.55 billion in 2030 and 9.74 billion in 2050. By 2100, the projected population will be 10.875 billion. [39]. In the context of the KSA, the population in 2019 was 34.27 million, and is estimated to reach 39.32 million by 2030. This population is projected to increase to 44.56 million in 2050 and reach 42.23 million in 2100 [39]. Table 3.1 shows the world and the KSA population.

TABLE 3.1 Projection of the world population.

	Population (millions)			
Major area	**2019**	**2030**	**2050**	**2100**
World	7,713	8,548	9,735	10,875
Africa	1,308	1,688	2,489	4,280
Asia	4,601	4,974	5,290	4,719
Europe	747	741	710	629
Latin America and the Caribbean	648	706	762	679
Northern America	366	390	425	490
Oceania	42	47	57	74
Saudi Arabia	34.269	39.322	44.562	42.231

Source: World Population Prospects 2019: Volume I. [110].

3.2.1 World ageing population

The ageing of the population is defined as *"more people living for longer compared with low birth of children"* [40]. The basis for defining elderly people varies, and the definitions can be categorized into three categories: (1) chronology, (2) change in social role, and (3) change in capabilities. The chronological age is the most common system in practice, as outlined by the World Health Organization (WHO).The United Nations defines elderly people as *"people 60 years old and above"* [41]. However, in many countries with high incomes, elderly people are those whose age is over 65, and consequently this is their age of qualification for social security benefits [42]. In this work we refer to elderly people as those who are 60+, according to the retirement policy in the KSA [9]. Most of the countries across the world are facing growth in the number of ageing population. The ageing population started increasing significantly in developed countries, and then, in the twenty-first century, this became a phenomenon in developing countries as well [8]. Globally, people aged 65 years and over comprised nearly 9% of the world population in 2019, with 702.9 million people. The number of elderly people in the world is projected to reach 1.55 billion in 2050 with an increase rate of 120% [43].

3.2.2 Ageing population in the KSA

The ageing population is a potentially major issue for the Government of the KSA, in respect of access to healthcare services. With the country experiencing growth in the economic and health sectors, the ageing population will incur health challenges if measures to address the situation are not taken into consideration [37,44]. The population of the KSA in 2015 was 31.5 million and is estimated to be 39.1 million in 2030 and this will increase to

46.1 million in 2050 and reach 47.6 million in 2100. The proportion of people aged below 15 years in the KSA has declined from 49.23% to 24.5% during the period from 1992 to 2019. It is expected that their number will drop to 18.7% in 2050 because of the reduction in fertility and mortality [45]. In contrast, the projections by the United Nations Department of Population estimate that the population of elderly people in the KSA is expected to increase. In 2019, the KSA ageing population was 1.169 million and this number is expected to reach 2.379 million by 2030 [43]. In particular, the number of elderly people in the KSA is increasing rapidly, from 5% of the total population in 2015 to a forecasted 20.9% by 2050. Among people who are aged more than 65 in the KSA, 79.4% of them receive treatment from chronic diseases through the government services provided in the healthcare centers, while 20.6% receive treatment at their own expenses. In addition, 70.5% of them suffering from physical movement difficulties, 24.2% have sight problems, and 5.3% are having hearing difficulties [46].

3.2.3 The impact of an ageing population

The ageing population presents many challenges for the world and the increased life expectancy and the reduction in the birth rate have many consequences, which can be clarified as follows.

3.2.3.1 Economy

3.2.3.1.1 Pensions

The lower rate of mortality applies to all age groups and, over time, feeds larger numbers into the ageing group. The increased (and still increasing) life expectancy increases the number of years people survive in the ageing group, and the number of people reaching very old ages. Both aspects have a great influence on pensions and on healthcare. The effects on pensions have created a crisis situation worldwide, for both governments and private pension schemes. The increasingly ageing population causes an increasing pressure on governments to provide and finance appropriate retirement benefit schemes. As a result of the growing numbers of beneficiaries, and of the fact that they draw their benefits for a much longer time than expected and budgeted years before, there is a need to increase the reserves of social security benefit to ensure that the amount of money available is sufficient to provide for all the beneficiaries. The governments also need to ensure that the funding is sustainable, and they need to set up appropriate measures to ensure continued availability of the benefits, as this "will not be a one-time need" requirement. Therefore, this will affect government budgets, as they need to allocate larger amounts to the retirement benefit scheme. This means that further contributions will need to be taken from taxpayers as they are the main sources of government revenue [7, 47–50].

In the KSA, the ageing population will increase pressure on government debt and public finance over the coming decades [51]. As the proportion of elderly people (above 60 years) increases, there will be more people eligible for pension benefits [10]. In 2015, the total number of employees at age 60 years and above was 160,860 thousand [52]. The retirement age is determined by the Saudi Government as 60 years. However, employees are now allowed to continue to work after they reach 60 years of age. The Public Pension Agency (PPA) calculates the benefits according to the years of service, which, to get full retirement benefits, should be 40 years worked before reaching 60 years of age. The PPA deducts 9% from employees' payroll during their working life. The normal retirement pension can be calculated as the number of worked years before the age of 60 multiplied by 1/40th of the final salary of the retiree, when he/she is eligible for retirement benefit. Particular regulations apply to people retiring for special reasons, for example, health [53]. In 2015, the total number of retirees was 710,672, which includes all cases of retirement, of which 532,117 are alive and 178,555 are deceased. The total amount that was paid by the government to the retirees or their dependents was Saudi Riyal (SR) 54,897 million in 2015, and the total amount that has been paid since the establishment of the PPA is SR 561,185 million [52].

3.2.3.1.2 Workforce

Elderly people, in some cases, require people to take care of them, especially if their age and health has affected their mobility. In these circumstances, caregivers are assigned to support them, either at their homes or at social care homes, and, therefore, new job opportunities are created for the workforce. Research worldwide shows that the number of those above 65 years will double by 2030, meaning that there will be more demand for caregivers [49, 54]. Therefore, in the KSA there is a need to fill the gaps, by 2030, in the nurse shortage with 100,000 more nursing positions, and, overall, 710,000 more healthcare professionals [55]. In the KSA, the ageing population (over 60 years) will significantly rise to 20.9% in 2050, which will lead to a decrease in the number of working people and could result in wage inflation. Furthermore, the total Labour Force Participation Rate is expected to fall from 53% in 2010 to 48.6% in 2050 [10]. This will cause shortages in all sectors of activity but will be particularly acute in the healthcare sector. One of the biggest challenges facing Saudi healthcare providers is the shortage of local healthcare professionals, such as pharmacists, nurses, and physicians. The majority of the health workforce are immigrants [56, 57]. In 2015, the total number in the health workforce was 282,865 employees; 86,756 physicians (26% Saudi), 23,626 pharmacists (21% Saudi), and 172,483 nursing staff (38.3 % Saudi) [58].

3.2.3.2 Healthcare

The increase in life expectancy will result in increasing healthcare costs per person: as people get older, they need more healthcare supports. Elderly people are susceptible to a number of illnesses and infections, as a result of weak bodies and immune systems. This results in the ageing population requiring more investment in healthcare to support them. According to a report by the WHO, by 2030, 60% of those above 65 years of age will be affected by one chronic disease. Despite the significant increase in the proportion of elderly people, the healthcare system is not currently designed to address the increasing demand for providing appropriate healthcare services for their needs [7, 48, 49, 59]. In the KSA, as a result of the ageing population increase, the expenditure on healthcare will grow as well [10].

3.2.3.3 *Family*

As people become older, in some cases they are no longer able to live alone, provide for themselves, or do certain things, such as cooking, shopping, etc., because of their increased inability to move around. In many cases, this burden is shifted to their relatives, and, therefore, their families have to spend extra money and time taking care of them. Thus, a changing population structure has created more responsibilities for families, with the consequent need to work more, to meet this extra duty [7, 49, 50]. In the Middle East and North Africa (MENA) region, the total population has increased, which has led to an increase in the ageing population. Therefore, the family structures and options for the care of elderly people will change [60]. In the KSA, the most common situation is that the oldest son/daughter takes care of their parents, although this is not always the case. The second most common option for wealthy children is to hire staff to take care of their family. A third option, for poor children is that they may apply for financial support to provide their parents with their needs. A fourth option is that nongovernmental organizations can provide support for elderly people. Lastly, the government can accommodate elderly people in social care homes and provide them with an acceptable quality of life [61]. The KSA Ministry of Health (MOH) currently provides 33,813 beneficiaries with social home healthcare from 180 hospitals [62]. A study has indicated that the majority of people who benefit from social home healthcare are the elderly, to be provided with a good quality of life [63]. Unfortunately, to the best of our knowledge, there are no statistical data about the family roles regarding their elderly relatives.

3.2.3.4 *Consumer spending*

As a result of changing needs due to changing population structure, consumer-spending is also changing. This is because customers of different age groups demand different types of goods and services. Consequently, consumer spending for consumables is affected by changes in the consumers' age structure and particularly by the larger percentage of people in the ageing population [64, 65]. In the KSA, elderly people have traditionally saved less and consumed more, due to their needs and lifestyle [10] as people get older, many of them are, sentimentally and for other reasons, attached to the house/apartment where they have lived for many years and do not want to move to a smaller one, even after their grown-up children have moved away and formed new households. Consequently, with the growing percentage of people in the ageing population and with important change in the housing market result on average a smaller number of inhabitants per house/apartment, and hence the need/demand for more houses/apartments to be built. Coupled with the additional housing needed for immigrants and for young people moving to larger towns, it has created a housing problem, fast increasing house prices, and even a crisis situation, in several countries [66].

3.2.4 Healthcare in the KSA

The KSA is the largest country in the Arabian Peninsula. The population of the KSA is 31 million, and the capital city is Riyadh, with a population of 7.7 million as of 2015 [67]. The desert dominates more than half the total area of the KSA [68].The MOH in the KSA is the main provider of healthcare services. The MOH provides Primary Health Care (PHC) facilities and services throughout a network of healthcare centers. The Saudi government provides citizens and residents with free access to health services through the public sector. The health system consists of three levels: primary, secondary, and tertiary healthcare. In addition, there are some private hospitals, where citizens have to pay for e-treatment [56, 69, 70] or which can be covered by their employers [71]. According to the Ministry of Health (2017) [110]), the KSA has experienced extensive growth in its healthcare system through improvements in staff training, quality of care, and integration of modern technology in the health sector. From 1970 to 2019, the KSA has increased its number of hospitals from 74 to 478. In 2015, the number of beds in the MOH was 41,297 in 274 hospitals. This accounts for 58.5% of hospitals, and the remainder are governmental (11,449) and private sector (16,648). The total number of PHC centers was 2282 across the country [58]. The government actual expenditure in 2018 was SR 175 billion (US $46.6 billion) for healthcare and social development. In 2019 and 2020, the government allocated SR 174 billion (US $46.4 billion) and SR 167 billion (US $44.5), respectively, for healthcare and social development [72].

Despite the massive budget allocated to the health sector by the Saudi Government, there are challenges in the provision of health services in the KSA. Some of these challenges can be summarized as: health workforce [56, 57, 69]; rapid increase in expenditure; pilgrim services; about 5 million pilgrims every year; [69]; health insurance; privatization of hospitals; diversifying financial sources [56]; language; cultural effects and prevalence of chronic diseases [57]. However, in 2016, the Saudi Government announced its "National transformation program 2020" which includes some initiatives by the MOH, which is planning to invest more than SR 23 billion in its new initiatives to achieve its "vision 2030" [73].The Ministry of Labour and Social Development is accountable for taking care of elderly people (aged over 60 years) who are unable to live independently and are not supported by their family. The Social Care Home is a department of the Ministry of Labour and Social Affairs, and its role is to provide elderly people with quality of life, including full healthcare for those who cannot be accommodated by their families. Currently, there are 12 social care homes in the KSA, which are located in Riyadh, Madinah, Makkah, Abha, Taif, Damam, Onizah, Jouf, and Wadi Al Dawasir [74].

3.3 AgeinginKSA website

The major concern for designing a website is to determine the purpose of building it [75]. Therefore, the purpose of building the website was to share knowledge with anyone interested in ageing in the KSA, to make the community aware of ageing in the KSA, to investigate the needs of elderly people, to assist elderly people to choose technology suitable for them, and to provide them with online training materials. This website is called AgeinginKSA and is based on a conceptual model AAL to provide a Home PMS (AALHPMS) [19] for the development of the AgeinginKSA website process.

The web portal will require that the homes of elderly persons be equipped with a set of sensors based on their needs, such as temperature sensors, emotion sensors, cameras (activation will depend on individual elders' authority), etc. The most important concerns for the model on existing homes are that they are cost efficient, and that the sensors can be retrofitted in a cost-effective way. The sensors should be installed easily, be flexible to be updated, and not require remodeling of the home. Obviously, this would not be significant concern for new builds as this would be addressed within the building control regulations to support AAL. Thus, the sensors will be positioned on walls, doors, floors, ceilings, and furniture. Furthermore, the elderly person can wear some of these appliances, such as the Smart watch, using wireless technology that makes retrofitting elderly persons' homes feasible. To assist in addressing the problems of the ageing population, which are rising in the KSA, a conceptual model was developed for supporting AALHPMS in the KSA [19]. The architecture of the model includes six layers briefly outlined as follows:

1. Data acquisition and processing (DAP) layer is the process of transferring signals, such as from heartbeat, motion sensors, etc., into a format that can be read [76]. Most of the devices are equipped with Smart sensors that enable devices to be connected to each other [77]. Therefore, DAP is responsible for collecting real-time data from different input sensors with different formats. The data are captured from elderly people in accordance with the specification and

instrumentation of each sensor, such as a Smart watch that measures heart rate. The Smart watch used would be a medically approved device appropriate for this application supplied by reputable vendors to strict medical specification. The data are transmitted via Bluetooth technology, or any wireless technologies that can support the connection. Then they are synchronized by using a mobile app, or by using a computer with installed connectivity. The data can then be transferred wirelessly to a web portal.

2. Communication structure (CS) layer is the backbone of the developed conceptual model. The major role of the CS layer is to connect devices together and enable them to share data. For this iteration, the CS consists of four types of network: Bluetooth, wireless, ZigBee, and Internet. It requires the availability of the Internet, which will help upload the data from the Smart devices, such as a phone or a laptop, to the online portal, via the wireless network, and will connect the Smart devices with the sensors via Bluetooth.
3. Data integration (DI) layer is the combination of data silos from different sources, which then delivers a coherent and consistent valuable view of the data [78]. Therefore, the data for this developed model will be collected from different sensors installed in the home of the elderly person, including motion sensors, temperature sensors, Smart watch, etc. This layer integrates and combines different structures and formats of data retrieved from different sensors into the data hub. The data collection should be more efficient and consistent, as it is filtered, cleaned, and uploaded to the hub. The process of DI consists of four types of databases: lifestyle, motion, and sensor databases, and (subject to the elderly person approval) an imagery database. This layer is responsible for storing and saving all applications and software into a hub. The hub can be a warehouse that integrates different data and converts them to valuable and meaningful information. The information can then be processed through the knowledge-reasoning layer using a rule-based expert system.
4. Cloud computing (CC) layer provides the computing resources through the Internet. CC allows the conceptual model to store and share the applications, software, processing resources, and data to Smart devices. The significant advantages of CC are the cost saving and the increases in service efficiency [79, 80]. The annual IT budget of an organization can be reduced by 10%–20% when shifting to CC [81]. This layer is the primary layer that connects the DI layer with the reasoning layer.
5. Knowledge reasoning (KR) layer uses a rule-based system that will assist in making proactive decisions. It processes and analyses large amounts of data and translates them into information and knowledge using, for example, SECI model of knowledge creation [82]. A KBS

can be used to transfer knowledge to resolve issues and problems [83]. It can also produce intelligent actions, using rule-based reasoning. Rule-based reasoning is considered to be the foundation of KBS [84]. Rule-based reasoning is responsible for collecting solutions based on the data [85, 86] acquired from different sensors. The information from AALHPMS can be used to provide proactive solutions that support medical actions.

6. Proactive control Centre (PCC) layer monitors the system and predicts and knows what type of issues and problems could happen to the elderly person, thereby supporting appropriate actions that are tailored to the specific problems. The actions that can be provided by PCC are: calling; texting; alerting and emailing the elderly; contacting families; contacting relatives or carers; visualizing daily activities; early reporting to families, relatives, carers, etc.; dispatching a doctor or a nurse and calling an ambulance and/or police.

AAL technology is a new concept in the KSA, and to the best of our knowledge, there are no studies that have investigated its use in the KSA to address the ageing population's challenges and issues. Elderly persons are very vulnerable to health issues. In some cases, instead of reacting after something has occurred, it is important to step back and be proactive, by monitoring the health of the elderly. It is extremely important to prevent the need for medical intervention, as well as ensuring it when it becomes necessary. Therefore, the developed web portal needs to be both responsive and proactive using dashboard interface for the PCC Layer.

3.3.1 PCC—the dashboard

In real life, people favor graphics, maps, visuals, and charts that present realistic views of the information [87]. The proposed system takes real-time information and from it delivers knowledge that is shown as patterns. The knowledge is generated by KR, which translates the integrated data into meaningful visualizations. It provides insights to the users. The system's visualization can be seen and monitored by a mobile, laptop, or any Smart devices. It is considered a value-added service, especially for the elderly person's family, relatives, and healthcare providers. This layer is used for visualizing the data received from sensors and stored in the Cloud. Eventually, visualization assists us in making representations that express a story about the data. Elderly people are subject to physical and mental issues. Their health is completely different from when they were younger, and health is a very complex process. Therefore, health problems might happen suddenly and accidentally. Sometimes, taking action after things have happened is not effective. Thus, instead of reacting when something occurs, it is extremely important to step back, and be proactive by monitoring the health of elderly people, and thus preventing the need for medical actions. The objective of the PCC dashboard is to ease the communication and monitoring process; in addition, it utilizes the data analysis to provide visualized outputs that are easy to understand [88, 89] which helps to predict the type of issues, and problems that could happen to the elderly person. Business Intelligence dashboards are effective tool for visualizing data to decision makers in the real time [89, 90].

The process of developing business intelligence dashboards encompasses six steps [91]; these steps are discussed for the purpose of PCC as follows:

1. *Setting the objectives*: The objective of PCC dashboard is to monitor elderly people and provide proactive notification and support escalation procedures when there is a problem, mainly if the heart rate drops under the minimum level. In addition, it should describe the location of the elderly person clearly and make access information of the elder or near relative and/or key holder much easier by screen sharing via Smart phones.
2. *Defining tasks, competencies, and responsibilities*: Doctors who are responsible for monitoring the elders will be able to track elders' location and monitor their heart rate and their current location. In the case of emergency, they will be able to know that intervention that would be needed and call near relative if appropriate.
3. *Setting the indicators*: Elders heart rate and location are constantly monitored through the dashboard.
4. *Collect data based on indicators*: Smart sensors and wearable devices as described in DAP layer will gather needed data for monitoring.
5. *Develop the dashboard*: The dashboard will be integrated into the website to allow the monitoring of each elder and being informed about the elders' current location.
6. *Evaluate the dashboard*: The dashboard should be evaluated in terms of understanding whether or not it achieves the intended development to support proactive monitoring of elderly people.

A PCC consists of a dashboard that has the functions of a PMS (PMS). The prototype PMS will assist in predicting the type of issues and problems that could occur in monitoring elderly persons based on KR, thereby supporting appropriate actions that are tailored to the specific problems for the individual. The multiscreen displays a dashboard that contains a map with location for each elderly person's details, the heart rate for a given period of time, the elderly person's location, and lifestyle and overall condition as shown in Fig. 3.1.

Monitoring an elderly person requires them first to register in PMS by following the operational processes described in Fig. 3.2.

The services that can be delivered to elderly people include: calling; texting, alerting and emailing the elderly person, contacting families, contacting relatives or carers; visualizing daily activities; early reports to

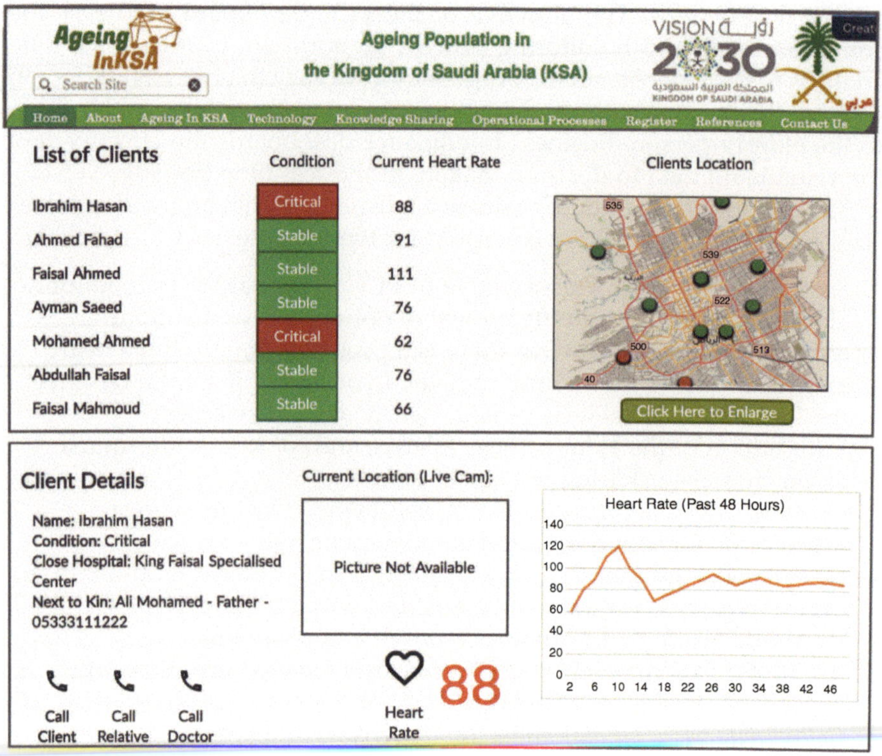

FIG. 3.1 The dashboard for monitoring an elderly person.

families, relatives, carers, etc.; dispatching a doctor or a nurse and calling an ambulance or the police. In the enhanced model, more sensors and networks can be added, based on the needs of the elderly person. Therefore, it is an agile conceptual model that can add or remove services based on the circumstances of elderly people.

3.3.2 Website development

Diffily [92] defined website development as a procedure for building a new website or applying changes to a live website, for instance adding an important new part to an existing website. This was named as website ageing in the KSA. The procedure for creating a website involves eight stages that can be described as follows:

- *Planning*: choose why you need a site and what to build
- *Content*: make a list of the substance you need
- *Design*: make an outline to show the substance
- *Construction*: compose the code and upload the material
- *Test*: ensure everything works appropriately

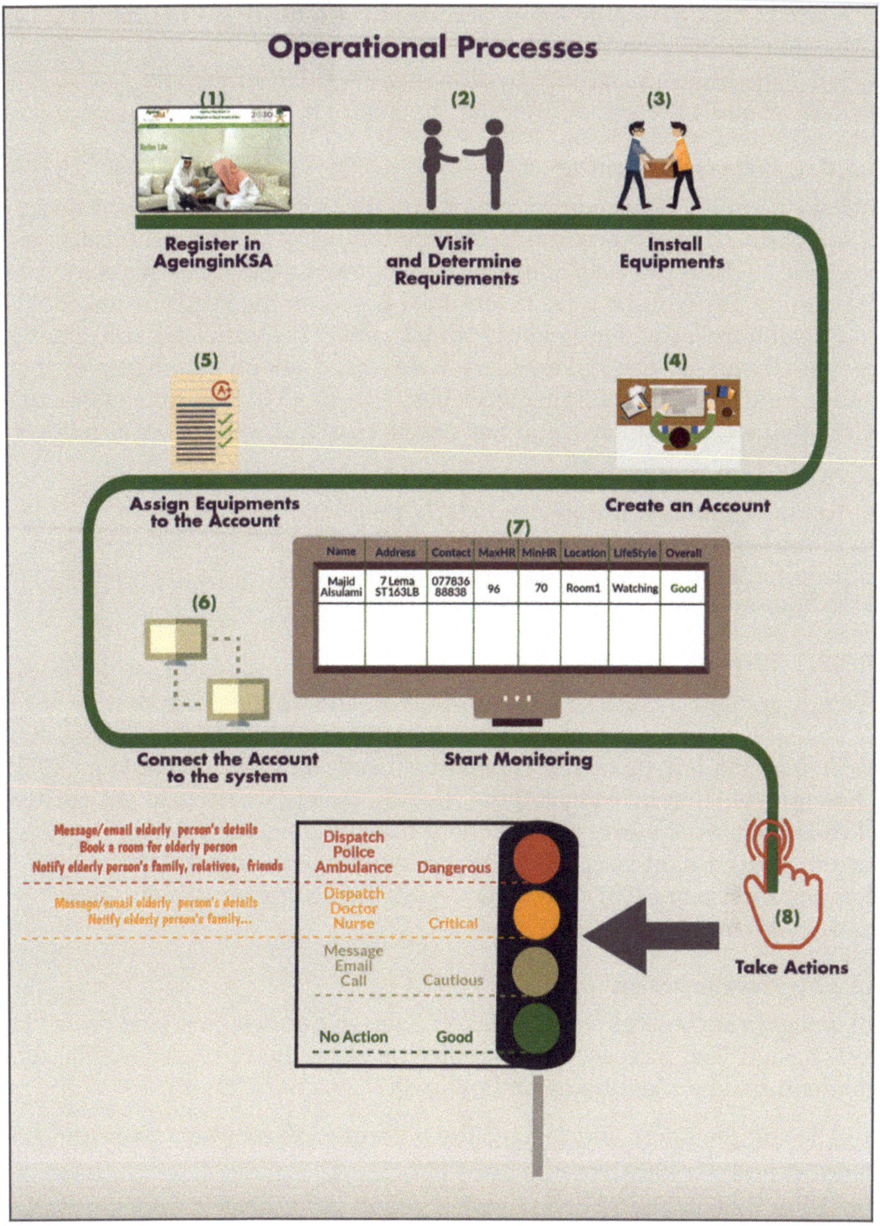

FIG. 3.2 The operational processes for PMS.

- *Hosting*: pick a domain name and discover a hosting provider to locate a website on the Internet
- *Publicity*: build up activity by drawing attention to the site
- *Review*: audit the site at intervals, to ensure it succeeds.

3.3.2.1 *Website planning*

Website planning is considered to be one of the important steps in the design of a website. It is a procedure to classify the users' needs and businesses' objectives, which can help start the development cycle [92]. The objectives of building this website were determined based on the needs of stakeholders: healthcare providers, elderly social care, IT specialists, and elderly people. Therefore, the stakeholders were asked about the objectives that should be achieved by building this website, through Community of Practice (CoP) that were conducted, and the objectives of this website are as follows:

- To make the community aware about ageing in the KSA
- To investigate the number of elderly people in the KSA
- To find solutions to assist elderly people in their daily activities and provide them with a better quality of life
- To investigate the needs of elderly people.

3.3.2.2 *Website content*

Website content includes most information and applications that need to be available online for AgeinginKSA. It was very important to ensure that most information provided meets the needs of the stakeholders [92]. Therefore, we first investigated the relevant ageing websites to get an idea of their content. We investigated these following ageing-related websites: http://www.asaging.org [93], http://www.ageuk.org.uk [94], http://aginginamerica.org [95], http://www.healthyageing.eu [96] and https://myageingparent.com [97].

3.3.2.2.3 Website design

To design a successful website, Jakob Nielsen defined "*ten good deeds*" in web design that increase the usability of virtually all websites. The ten elements can be identified as follow [98]:

- Allocate the name and logo of the organization on every page and hyperlink the logo to the home page
- Add a search engine
- Describe the headlines and page titles as simply as possible
- Build the page so as to simplify scanning
- Use hypertext to structure the content space
- Display product photos
- Use relevance-enhanced image reduction
- Use link titles

- Ensure that all essential pages are accessible for users with disabilities
- Adopt what the best websites do in an appropriate technique.

A study conducted by Al-salebi [99] indicated that there must be three significant features to make a good website. These features initiate four attributes of the website, which can be defined as personalization, responsiveness, interactivity, and contrast and the three features are as follows: first, visual design is an important feature in the design of a good website. This feature depends on five issues, which are page layout, navigation, consistency, embedding pictures or flashes, and using appropriate colors. Second, readability is considered as an essential feature for making a readable website. This feature depends on three issues, which are font size, font family, and font color. Third, content can be identified as the added value of the website. This feature depends on six issues that are original content, credible content, grammar and structure of content, breaking the text's content into paragraphs, clean content, and search engine.

To design a good website, designers should take into consideration some of the usability problems that may lead to failure. Therefore, it is important to evaluate the severity of web usability problems systematically [100]. This can assist the designers to overcome these issues at the beginning of the project of website designing. Nielsen and Loranger [100] outlined in their book the most important factors that cause the failure of websites, which are as follows:

- Search tools
- Findability (Information architecture, category names, navigation, links)
- Page design (readability, layout, graphics, amateur, scrolling)
- Information (content, product info, corporate info, prices)
- Task support (workflow, privacy, forms, comparison, inflexibility)
- Fancy design (multimedia, back button, PDF/printing, new window, sound)
- Others (bugs, presence on web, ads, new site, metaphors).

3.3.2.3 *Website construction*

Website construction is a procedure for translating design and content into code [92]. We used a wix.com, which is a *"leading cloud-based development platform with millions of users worldwide."* It has many templates that allow anyone to build a professional website easily [101]. Therefore, we did not need to write any codes to construct the design and contents. Diffily [92] indicated that browser compatibility and screen resolution are very important for the website to be compatible with best practice. Thus, AgeinginKSA was tested on Internet Explorer, Firefox, Safari, and Google Chrome. The AgeinginKSA used 1024 pixels wide and 768 pixels high for the screen resolution and was designed to be compatible with mobiles.

3.3.2.4 Website test

Website testing is considered to be the process used to evaluate the website, based on the guideline agreements. It ensures that the website meets the minimum standards to achieve its goal and objective [92]. We have run many tests for AgeinginKSA.org using different website testers such as:

- www.website.grader.com showing that the overall average for testing AgeinginKSA.org is 84 of 100.
- Using www.nibbler.silktide.com the accessibility criterion indicated that it scored 9 of 10, while the technology scored 8.5 of 10.
- www.pingdom.com presented a good performance with a grade of 80 of 100.
- www.powermapper.com proved that AgeinginKSA.org is compatible with most of the well-known browsers, and also with mobiles' browsers. It reported that there are no issues.
- www.search.google.com/test/mobile-friendly indicated that AgeinginKSA.org is designed to be mobile-friendly.
- www.checkmycolours.com tested the colors used in AgeinginKSA.org, and reported no issues related to them.

3.3.2.5 Website hosting

Website hosting is a space in which the website is stored and can be accessed via the Internet [92]. Wix.com is the hosting provider that was chosen for the website, and the domain name is ageingingksa.org. We selected .org because AgeinginKSA is a nonprofit organization.

3.3.2.6 Website publicity

The website was disseminated via a series of social communications, such as Twitter, Facebook, LinkedIn, and using Instant Messages such as WhatsApp. In addition, Wix.com provides search engine optimization (SEO).

3.3.2.7 Website review

According to the website's plan, reviewing the website indicates that the goal and objectives have been accomplished.

3.3.3 An overview of the AgeinginKSA website

At the first stage, AgeinginKSA was designed in the English language, and then, according to the results of the focus group that was held for the evaluation session and following requests to translate AgeinginKSA into the Arabic language, the Arabic website was designed covering the English and Arabic languages. In the following sections, we explain the contents of AgeinginKSA.

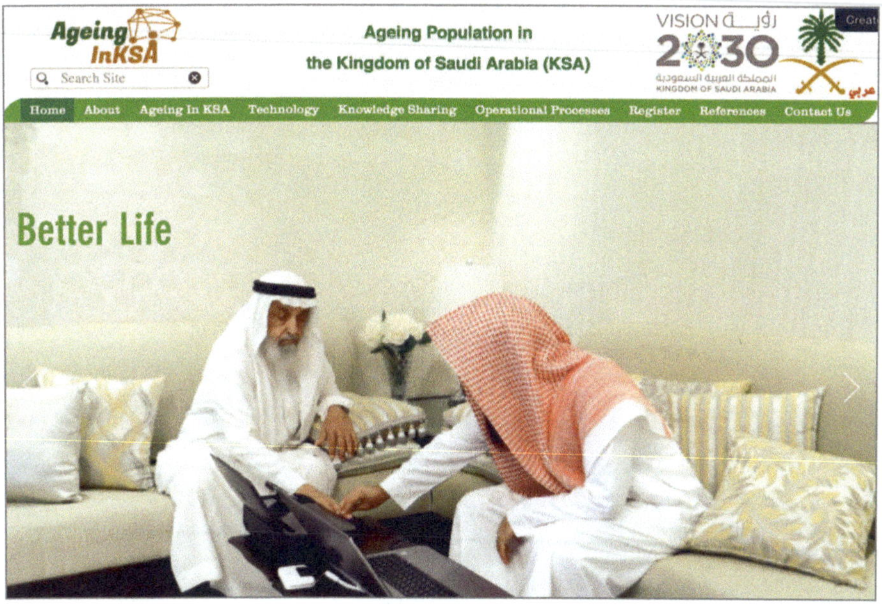

FIG. 3.3 English home page of AgeinginKSA.

3.3.3.1 *Home page of AgeinginKSA*

A home page is considered the main page of a website that is navigated by users. It assists users to move between other pages in AgeinginKSA. It consists of a logo in the left corner, search engine, title of the website, and the vision 2030 of Saudi Arabia. It has many pages, which are about ageing in the KSA, technology, social media, registration, references, and contacts. Fig. 3.3 shows the English home page and Fig. 3.4 illustrates the Arabic home page. It contains a slideshow with six images that reflect the meaning of ageing.

The second part of the main page, which includes the contact number and email and the twitter account, is shown in Fig. 3.5.

3.3.3.2 *About page*

The about page is composed of three subpages: objectives, context, and team, as shown in Fig. 3.6. The objectives subpage is to clarify the purposes of the AgeinginKSA website, which are to collaborate with ministries, researchers, healthcare providers, elderly people, families, and related organizations and people, in order:

- To make the community aware about ageing in the KSA
- To investigate the number of elderly people in the KSA
- To find solutions to assist elderly people in their daily activities and provide them with a better quality of life
- To investigate the needs of elderly people.

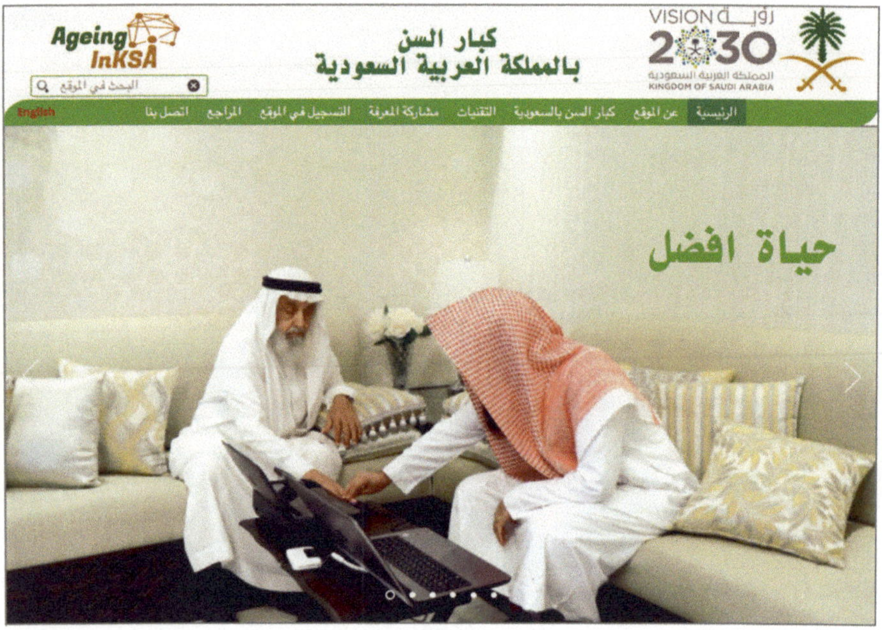
Ageing InKSA
البحث في الموقع
كبار السن
بالمملكة العربية السعودية
VISION رؤية
2030
المملكة العربية السعودية
KINGDOM OF SAUDI ARABIA
English
اتصل بنا
المراجع
التسجيل في الموقع
مشاركة المعرفة
التقنيات
كبار السن بالسعودية
عن الموقع
الرئيسية
حياة افضل

FIG. 3.4 Arabic home page of ageing in KSA.

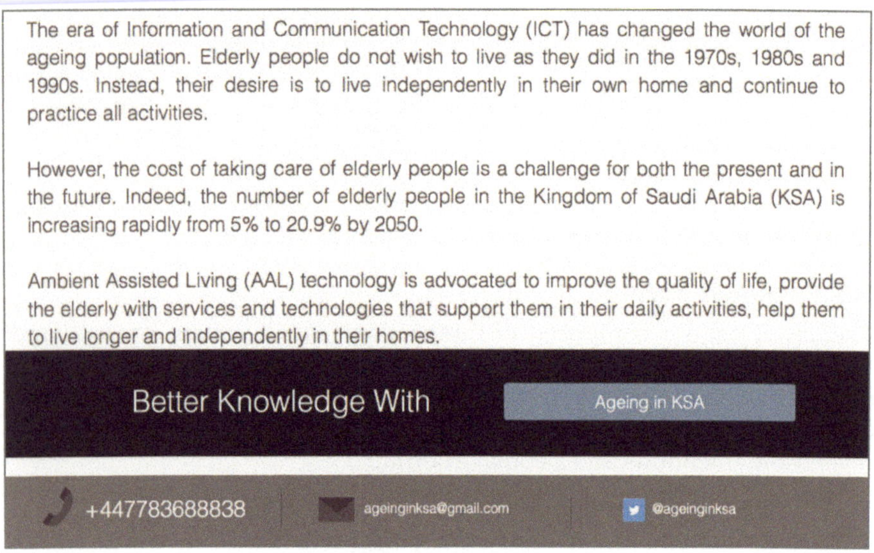
The era of Information and Communication Technology (ICT) has changed the world of the ageing population. Elderly people do not wish to live as they did in the 1970s, 1980s and 1990s. Instead, their desire is to live independently in their own home and continue to practice all activities.
However, the cost of taking care of elderly people is a challenge for both the present and in the future. Indeed, the number of elderly people in the Kingdom of Saudi Arabia (KSA) is increasing rapidly from 5% to 20.9% by 2050.
Ambient Assisted Living (AAL) technology is advocated to improve the quality of life, provide the elderly with services and technologies that support them in their daily activities, help them to live longer and independently in their homes.
Better Knowledge With
Ageing in KSA
+447783688838
ageinginksa@gmail.com
@ageinginksa

FIG. 3.5 The second part of main page.

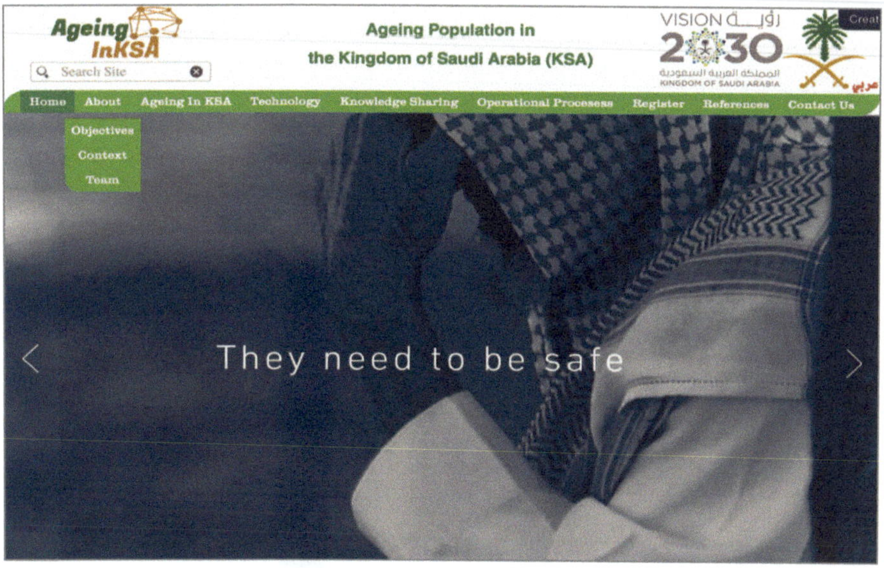

FIG. 3.6 About page of AgeinginKSA.

The context subpage presents the idea of designing AgeinginKSA, while the team subpage introduces a short resume of the website developers.

3.3.3.3 Ageing in KSA page

The ageing in KSA page is composed of two subpages, which includes ageing and causes of the ageing population, as illustrated in Fig. 3.7. The

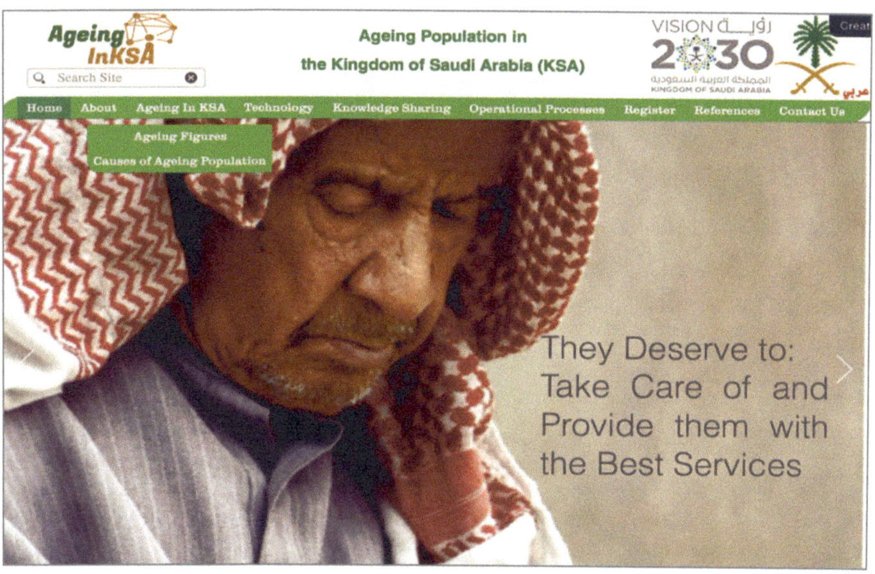

FIG. 3.7 Ageing in KSA page.

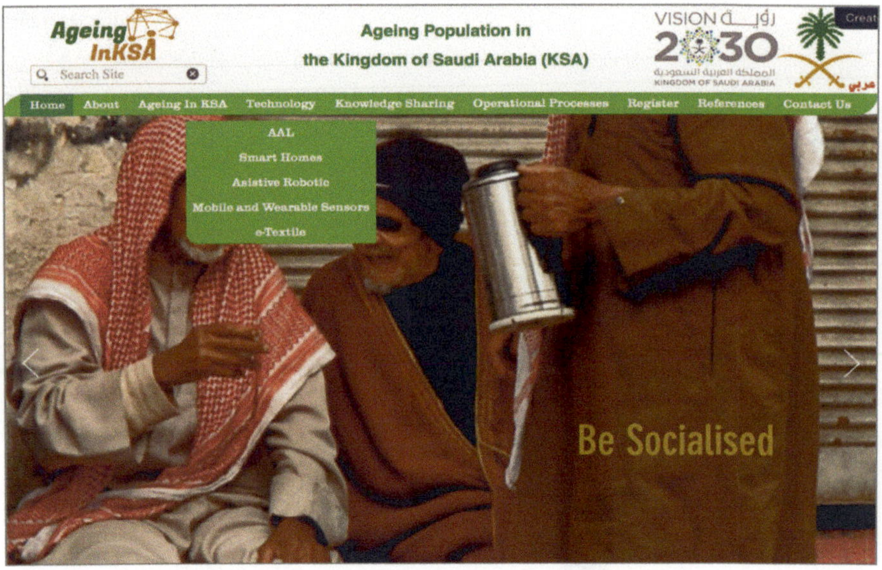

FIG. 3.8 Technology page.

ageing Fig's subpage presents some statistics about the ageing population in the KSA, and the second subpage indicates the causes of ageing, which are fertility, mortality, and international immigration.

3.3.3.4 Technology page

This page contains five subpages and explains AAL technologies, which are Smart homes, Assistive robotics, Mobile and Wearable sensors, and e-Textiles as seen in Fig. 3.8.

3.3.3.5 Knowledge sharing page

Many technological tools can be used to share knowledge. This page describes the tools that we used on the website, as illustrated in Fig. 3.9.

3.3.6 Operational processes page

This page explains the processes to subscribe in the monitoring system that we proposed. Fig. 3.10 presents the suggested processes.

3.3.3.7 Registration page

This page consists of a form that allows people to register with the website to subscribe to the monitoring system, as shown in Fig. 3.11.

3.3.3.8 References page

This page contains all references for the images that have been used, and the references for the contents of the website, as shown in Fig. 3.12.

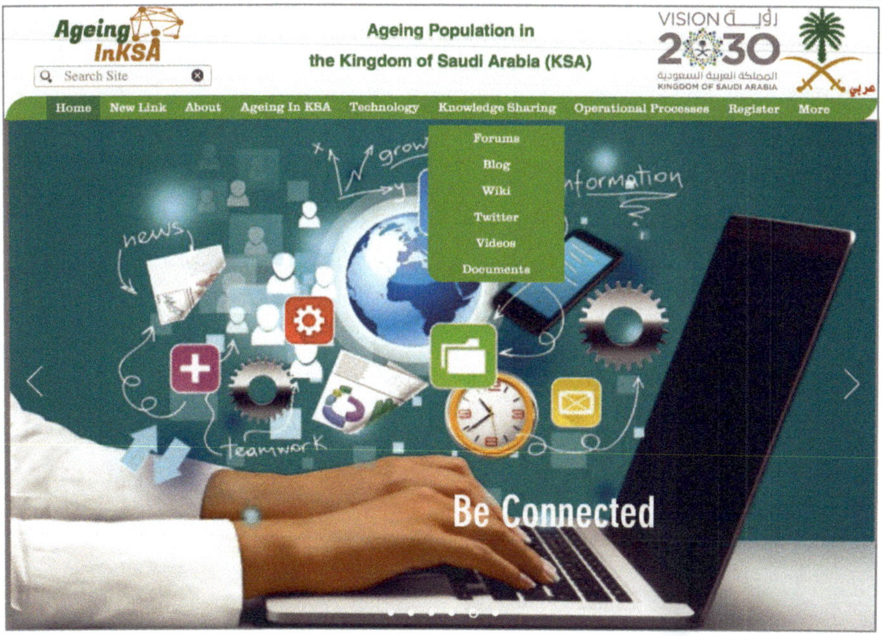

FIG. 3.9 Knowledge sharing page.

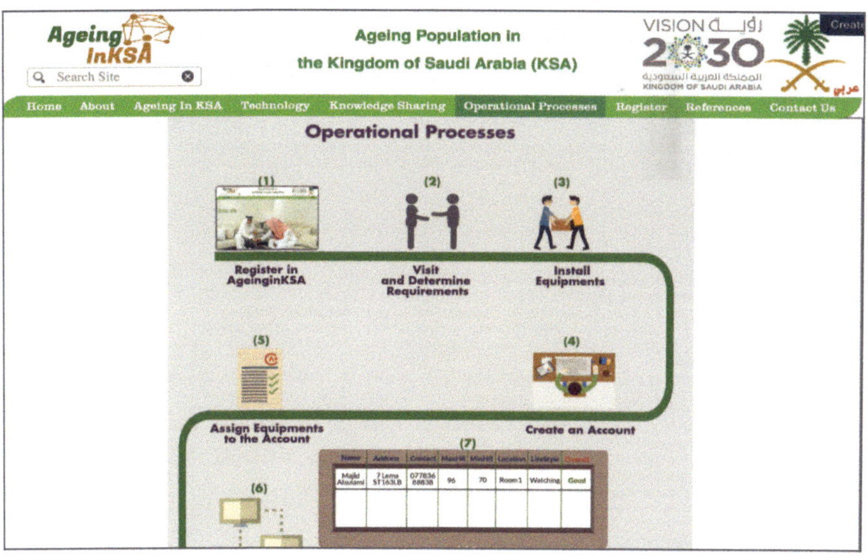

FIG. 3.10 The operational processes for subscribing in the proposed monitoring system.

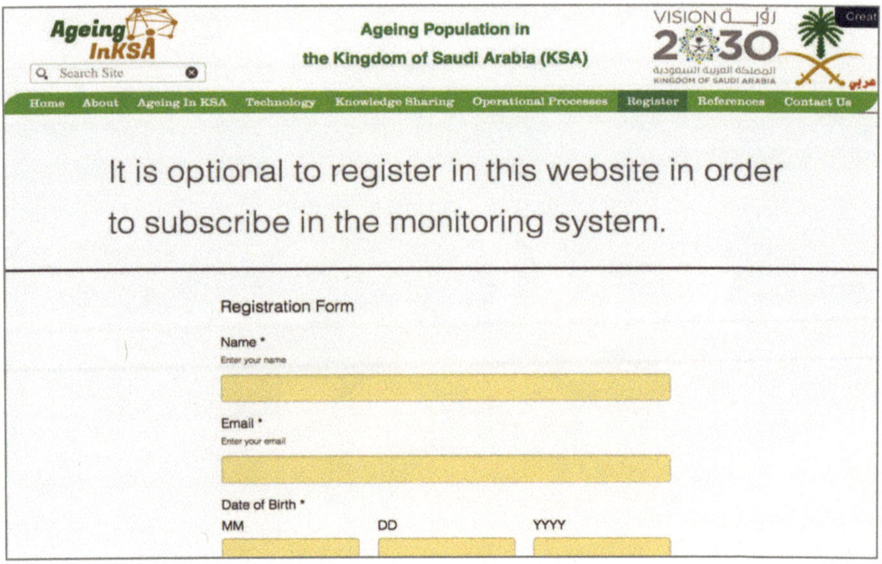

FIG. 3.11 Registration form.

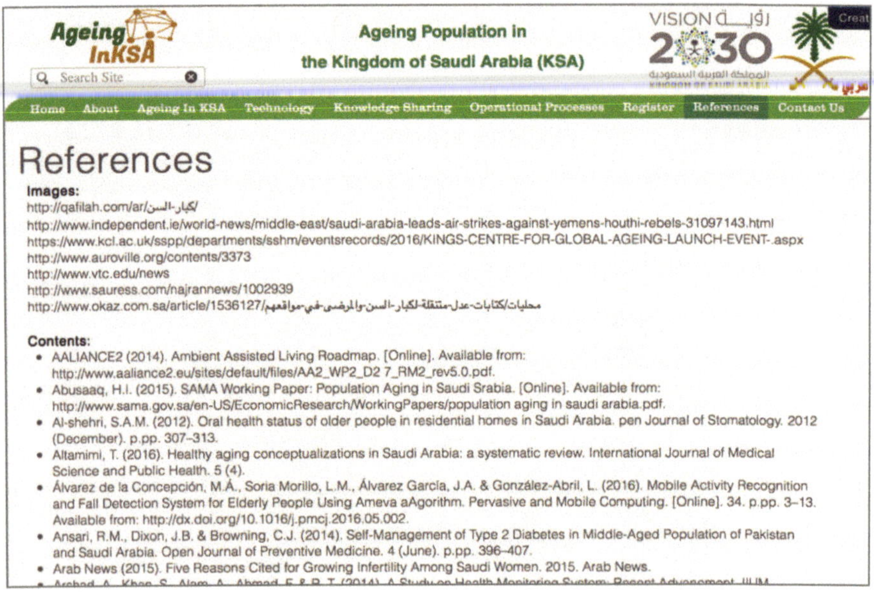
Ageing InKSA
Search Site
Ageing Population in
the Kingdom of Saudi Arabia (KSA)
VISION رؤية
2030
المملكة العربية السعودية
Home
About
Ageing In KSA
Technology
Knowledge Sharing
Operational Processes
Register
References
Contact Us
References
Images:
http://qafilah.com/ar/كبار-السن/
http://www.independent.ie/world-news/middle-east/saudi-arabia-leads-air-strikes-against-yemens-houthi-rebels-31097143.html
https://www.kcl.ac.uk/sspp/departments/sshm/eventsrecords/2016/KINGS-CENTRE-FOR-GLOBAL-AGEING-LAUNCH-EVENT-.aspx
http://www.auroville.org/contents/3373
http://www.vtc.edu/news
http://www.sauress.com/najrannews/1002939
http://www.okaz.com.sa/article/1536127/محليات/كتابات-عدل-متنقلة-لكبار-السن-والمرضى-في-مواقعهم
Contents:
• AALIANCE2 (2014). Ambient Assisted Living Roadmap. [Online]. Available from: http://www.aaliance2.eu/sites/default/files/AA2_WP2_D2 7_RM2_rev5.0.pdf.
• Abusaaq, H.I. (2015). SAMA Working Paper: Population Aging in Saudi Srabia. [Online]. Available from: http://www.sama.gov.sa/en-US/EconomicResearch/WorkingPapers/population aging in saudi arabia.pdf.
• Al-shehri, S.A.M. (2012). Oral health status of older people in residential homes in Saudi Arabia. pen Journal of Stomatology. 2012 (December). p.pp. 307–313.
• Altamimi, T. (2016). Healthy aging conceptualizations in Saudi Arabia: a systematic review. International Journal of Medical Science and Public Health. 5 (4).
• Álvarez de la Concepción, M.Á., Soria Morillo, L.M., Álvarez García, J.A. & González-Abril, L. (2016). Mobile Activity Recognition and Fall Detection System for Elderly People Using Ameva aAgorithm. Pervasive and Mobile Computing. [Online]. 34. p.pp. 3–13. Available from: http://dx.doi.org/10.1016/j.pmcj.2016.05.002.
• Ansari, R.M., Dixon, J.B. & Browning, C.J. (2014). Self-Management of Type 2 Diabetes in Middle-Aged Population of Pakistan and Saudi Arabia. Open Journal of Preventive Medicine. 4 (June). p.pp. 396–407.
• Arab News (2015). Five Reasons Cited for Growing Infertility Among Saudi Women. 2015. Arab News.

FIG. 3.12 References page.

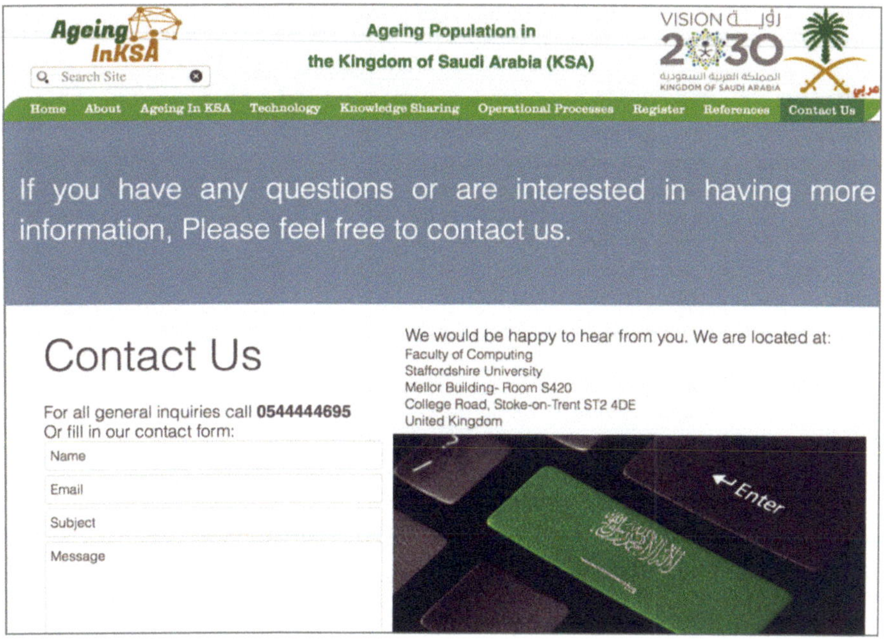
Ageing InKSA
Search Site
Ageing Population in
the Kingdom of Saudi Arabia (KSA)
VISION 2030
KINGDOM OF SAUDI ARABIA
Home About Ageing In KSA Technology Knowledge Sharing Operational Processes Register References Contact Us
If you have any questions or are interested in having more information, Please feel free to contact us.
Contact Us
For all general inquiries call 0544444695
Or fill in our contact form:
Name
Email
Subject
Message
We would be happy to hear from you. We are located at:
Faculty of Computing
Staffordshire University
Mellor Building- Room S420
College Road, Stoke-on-Trent ST2 4DE
United Kingdom
Enter

FIG. 3.13 Contact us page.

3.3.3.9 *Contact us page*

To ask for further help or more information about the website, a help page was designed and is outlined in Fig. 3.13.

3.3.4 Evaluation of the usability of the website AgeinginKSA

Evaluation can be defined as "*the process of determining the extent to which objectives have been attained*" [102]. Usability can be defined as "*a quality attribute that assesses how easy user interfaces are to use. The word "usability" also refers to methods for improving ease-of-use during the design process*" [103]. The usability evaluation process can be defined as "*an effective method by which a software development team can establish the positive and negative aspects of its prototype releases, and make the required changes before the system is delivered to the target users*" [104]. To evaluate the usability of the AgeinginKSA website, we used heuristic evaluation. This is considered an effective and efficient method to evaluate a website and identify usability problems [105, 106]. Therefore, we used the guidelines for heuristic evaluation that were proposed by Nielsen [107], and severity ratings for usability problems that was outlined by Nielsen [108], as shown in Table 3.2 with a rating scale from 0 to 4 for the following:

0 = I do not agree that this is a usability problem at all

1 = Cosmetic problem only: it does not need to be fixed, unless extra time is available on the project

TABLE 3.2 An instrument to evaluate AgeinginKSA website.

Heuristics	Statements	Rating scale				
		0	1	2	3	4
Visibility of system status	The AgeinginKSA can provide users with feedback while working on the website, within an appropriate time. (e.g., header explains screen contents, action when object is chosen, cursor points the selected item.)					
Match between system and the real world	AgeinginKSA uses terms familiar to users and information appears logical and natural. (e.g., Icons are familiar, menu in logical order)					
User control and freedom	AgeinginKSA provides users with freedom and control. (e.g., users can cancel any action; users can stop interacting at any time).					
Consistency and standards	AgeinginKSA is built to be consistent and standardized. (e.g., each window has a title, icons are labeled, menu names match the meaning)					
Error prevention	AgeinginKSA can address error handling. (e.g., the number of character spaces is presented in the text box, warning message shown when error occurs).					
Recognition rather than recall	AgeinginKSA offers instructions on how to use it. (e.g., name of pages).					
Flexibility and efficiency of use	AgeinginKSA is designed to be used by experienced and inexperienced users.					
Aesthetic and minimalist design	AgeinginKSA demonstrates relevant contents that are relevant to the stakeholder's needs.					
Help users recognize, diagnose, and recover from errors	AgeinginKSA provides error messages that can be used to advise and provide instructions for correction and recovery. (e.g., form of support)					
Help and documentation	AgeinginKSA provides help and documentation. It can be easily searched, and information is easily found. (e.g., form of support).					

2 = Minor usability problem: fixing this should be given low priority

3 = Major usability problem: important to fix it, so should be given high priority

4 = Usability catastrophic: imperative to fix this before the product can be released.

3.3.4.1 *Evaluation focus group in the KSA for website AgeinginKSA*

One of the significant advantages of carrying out a focus group is the richness and depth of information that can be gained and learned. The acceptable size for a focus group can be between 6 and 10 participants [109]. Therefore, a focus group was assembled in King Abdul Aziz University, Jeddah, Saudi Arabia to evaluate the AgeinginKSA website. Nine participants (three IT specialists, three healthcare providers, and three elderly people) attended, and the Arabic language was preferred. However, the presentation of the concept was written in the English language but was presented in Arabic and the sessions were recorded. The focus group was divided into two sessions as follows:

- The first session was an introduction to the AgeinginKSA website, and the session took 40 min
- The second session was about evaluating the AgeinginKSA website and this session took 60 min.

3.3.4.2 *Scenario of the evaluation*

The evaluation started in the second session. The researcher clarified the aims of the evaluation and the techniques to be used. The participants were provided with information and guidance to encompass ethical matters, such as the ability to withdraw from the survey at any time. The information relating to the AgeinginKSA website was online, and the relevant links were sent to the participants. The participants were able to use their phones to participate in the online information session.

3.3.4.3 *Demographic of the participants*

It was important to engage participants relevant to the concepts of the evaluation. Three groups of stakeholders were involved in this evaluation process for the AgeinginKSA website and as the site is related to elderly people; therefore, this age group was involved in the evaluation. The healthcare providers were considered as the second stakeholders, because they have responsibilities to support elderly people and provide for their needs. Finally, the IT specialists could implement the conceptual model and design websites.

All participants were selected carefully to make sure they had sufficient knowledge about evaluating the concepts of the developed system. The age group 20–40 years old made up 55.56% (five participants) of respondents, the age group 41–59 made up 11.11% (one participant), and 33.33% of respondents (three participants) were above 60 years old, as shown in Fig. 3.14.

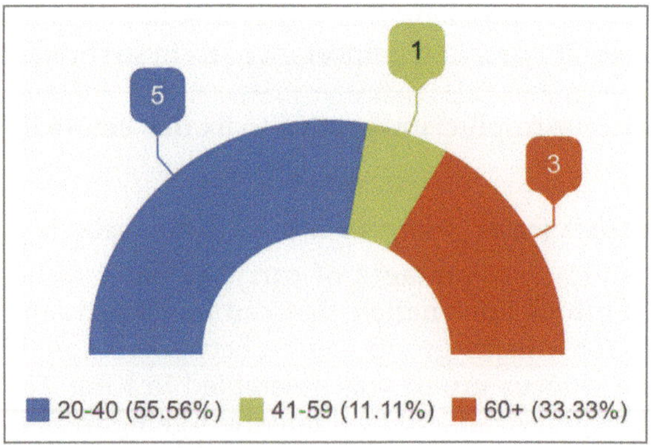

FIG. 3.14 Demographics of participants.

3.3.4.4 *AgeinginKSA evaluation*

In the second session, the 10 guidelines for heuristic evaluation, proposed by Nielsen [107], were used for the evaluation of AgeinginKSA. The evaluation instrument consisted of 10 statements, chosen to evaluate AgeinginKSA and to identify usability problems, with the addition of an open-ended question, which was *"Are there any other suggestions that you would like to add?"*

- Visibility of system status

  The results showed that most of the participants indicated that there are no problems with the visibility of the system status. A total of 89% of participants indicated that AgeinginKSA can provide users working on the website with feedback within an appropriate time, while only one elderly person (11%) indicated that AgeinginKSA has a cosmetic problem related to visibility.

- Match between the system and the real world

  A total of 89% of participants indicated that AgeinginKSA uses terms that are familiar to users, and that information appears logical and natural. This result emphasizes that AgeinginKSA was designed to match the real world. Only one elderly person (11%) indicated that AgeinginKSA has a cosmetic problem related to this statement.

- User control and freedom

  The majority of participants, 89%, reported that there are no issues with this factor, while one elderly person (11%) indicated that AgeinginKSA does not provide the user with freedom and control.

- Consistency and standards

  Eight participants (89%) reported that AgeinginKSA is built to be consistent and standardized, and it is easy to navigate. One elderly person (11%) indicated that AgeinginKSA has a cosmetic problem to be solved if possible.

- Error prevention

  This factor was evaluated positively by seven participants (78%) who indicated that AgeinginKSA can address errors when they happen. However, 22% of participants (two elderly people) mentioned that there is a cosmetic problem.
- Recognition rather than recall

  Eight participants (89%) reported that AgeinginKSA provides clear instructions on how to use every page, while 11% of participants (one elderly person) indicated it is missing some instructions and that changes should be made if time is available.
- Flexibility and efficiency of use

  Six of the participants (67%) indicated that AgeinginKSA can easily be used and no usability problems happened while exploring it. However, 33% of participants (two elderly people and one healthcare provider) reported that this factor has a minor problem.
- Aesthetic and minimalist design

  All participants (100%) reported that AgeinginKSA demonstrates having relevant contents regarding the ageing population in the KSA and the AAL technologies that can be used to provide elderly people with a good quality of life and services they need.
- Help for users to recognize, diagnose, and recover from errors

  AgeinginKSA provides users with forms that allow them to register with the website, and once an error occurs it notifies users. A total of 67% of participants indicated there is no usability problem with this factor, while 22% of participants reported that there is a cosmetic problem. In addition, 11% of participants stated there is a minor problem with this factor.
- Help and documentation

  Eight participants (89%) indicated that the AgeinginKSA provides help files and support forms to make it easy to find answers to any questions. One elderly person suggested that this factor should be fixed if extra time is available (11%).
- Overall AgeinginKSA evaluation

  The overall evaluation for AgeinginKSA for the 10 guidelines is 82%, which indicates there are no major problems with it. This indicates that AgeinginKSA has met the requirements of the stakeholders, which are elderly people, healthcare providers, and IT specialists, and showed that they are satisfied with the design of AgeinginKSA and its contents, as shown in Fig. 3.15.

3.3.4.5 *Suggestions*

Seven of the participants suggested that a translation of AgeinginKSA into the Arabic language should be done immediately. Another suggestion was about adding a Saudi mobile number to the "contact us" page. The final suggestion was about adding the Saudi 2030 vision logo and its link. The authors studied these suggestions carefully to ascertain whether they

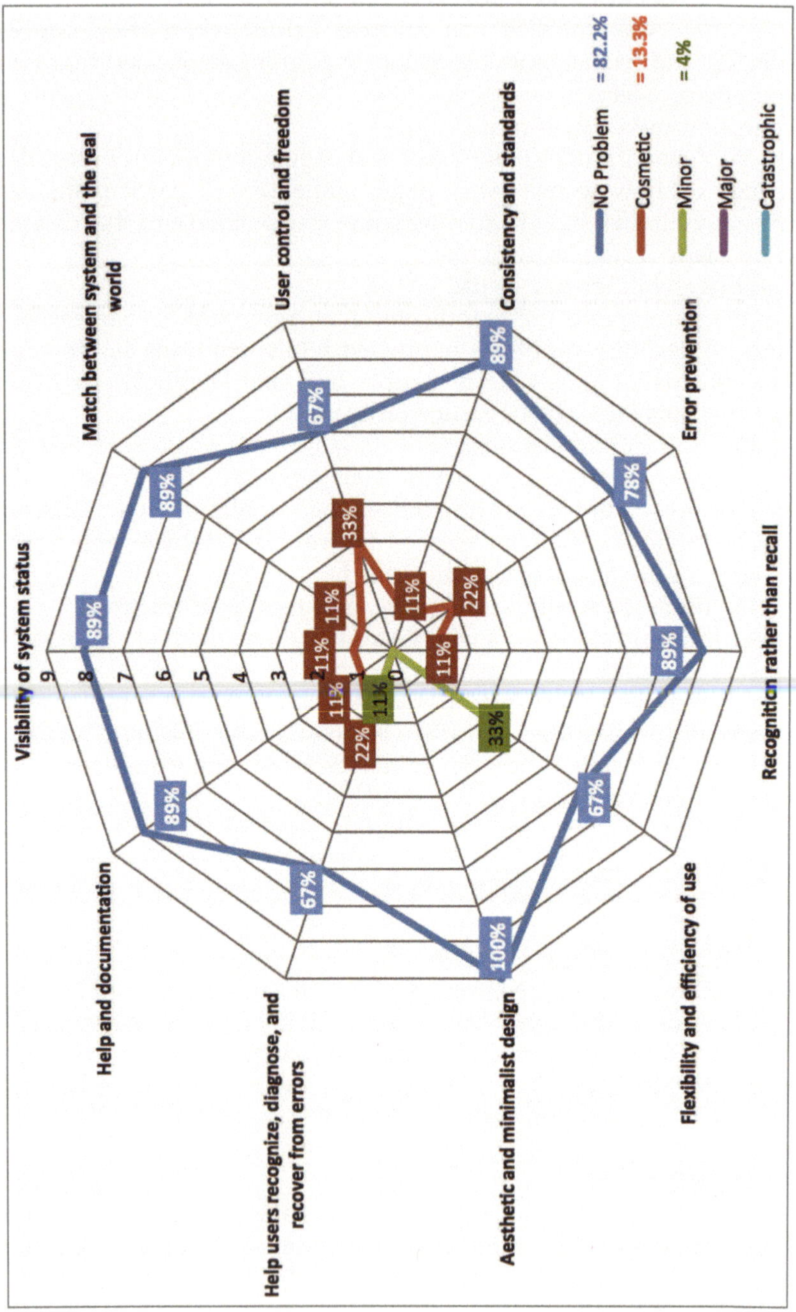

FIG. 3.15 Overall AgeinginKSA Evaluation.

would improve the website. Consequently, these three suggestions were accepted and incorporated into AgeinginKSA Website.

3.4 Conclusion

The chapter discusses the use of a conceptual AALHPMS to support elderly people in the KSA and the use of a web portal AgeinginKSA. The designed AAL dashboard used in the system allows the monitoring of elderly person and tracks their activity in the real time. The PCC dashboard is designed to display the data acquired from the sensors and Smart wearable devices (medically approved to specified standards by reputable vendors) by the elderly and also the accompanying AAL devices and technology installed in their homes. It allows displaying a live screen to check their current activity, heart rate, and other information related to elderly person. In the case of emergency, the controller can access the elderly person details immediately and initially call the client to check for "false alarm." If the client is unavailable this would necessitate the escalation of the emergency procedure to inform the next-to-kin and/or key holder and sharing the monitoring screens with them concerning location via Smart phone of the elderly person and placing health staff on standby. In addition, it would also allow calling the nearest hospital stored in the database, which contains the elderly person medical file. The AgeinginKSA website is designed to raise the knowledge on AAL technologies; and it allows elderly person to register for services to be able to be monitored through the dashboard and provide appropriate details needed for the monitoring process such as the address and phone number for the next-to-kin. The website describes different technologies used for the purpose of monitoring as well as allowing the elderly person to be in contact with the monitoring center through the web portal and provide feedback on the service provided. The intention in the future is that the web portal could be expanded allowing social interaction between elderly people coordinated by social services to improve community facilities and quality of life of the elderly citizens of KSA. AAL technology is a new concept in the KSA, and to the best of our knowledge, there are no studies investigating its use in the KSA to address the ageing population's challenges and issues.

References

[1] E.F.V.D. Isselt, et al., Geriatric rehabilitation in older patients with cardiovascular disease: a feasibility study, Eur. Geriatr. Med. 9 (6) (2018) 853–861. Available at https://link.springer.com/article/10.1007/s41999-018-0119-2.

[2] R. Sokullu, A. Balcı, E. Demir, The role of drones in ambient assisted living systems for the elderly, In: I. Ganchev, N.M. Garcia, C. Dobre, C.X. Mavromoustakis, R. Goleva (Eds.) Enhanced Living Environments: Algorithms, Architectures, Platforms, and Systems, Springer, Cham, 2019, pp. 295–321.

[3] R. Li, B. Lu, K.D. McDonald-Maier, Cognitive assisted living ambient system: a survey, Digit. Commun. Netw. Elsevier 1 (4) (2015) 229–252, doi:10.1016/j.dcan.2015.10.003.
[4] J.M. Corchado, J. Bajo, A. Abraham, GerAmi: improving healthcare delivery in geriatric residences, IEEE Intell. Syst. 23 (2) (2008) 19–25, doi:10.1109/MIS.2008.27.
[5] R.M. Ansari, J.B. Dixon, C.J. Browning, Self-management of type 2 diabetes in middle-aged population of Pakistan and Saudi Arabia, Open J. Prev. Med. 4 (2014) 396–407.
[6] R. Blasco, et al., A Smart kitchen for ambient assisted living, Sensors (Basel, Switzerland) 14 (2014) 1629–1653, doi:10.3390/s140101629.
[7] United Nations (2015a) World Population Ageing 2015 Report. https://www.un.org/en/development/desa/population/publications/pdf/ageing/WPA2015_Report.pdf.
[8] United Nations (2015b) World Population Ageing Highlights. https://www.un.org/en/development/desa/population/publications/pdf/ageing/WPA2015_Highlights.pdf [Accessed 5 May 2017].
[9] H.M. Alsufiani, et al., Dietary patterns, nutrient intakes, and nutritional and physical activity status of Saudi older adults: a narrative review, J. Aging Res. Clin. Pract. 4 (1) (2015) 2–11.
[10] H. I. Abusaaq, (2015) Population aging in Saudi Arabia. Economic Research Department, Saudi Arabian Monetary Agency, working Paper, WP/15/2.
[11] S.A.M. Al-Shehri, Oral health status of older people in residential homes in Saudi Arabia, Open J. Stomatol. 02 (04) (2012) 307–313, doi:10.4236/ojst.2012.24053.
[12] M. Moradi-Lakeh, et al., Self-medication with antibiotics: questionnaire survey among primary care center attendants, Pharmacoepidemiol. Drug Saf. 18 (12) (2015) 1150–1157, doi:10.1002/pds.
[13] H. Alruwaili, et al., Symptoms and risk for obstructive sleep apnea among sample of Saudi Arabian adults, Sleep Biol. Rhythms 13 (4) (2015) 332–341, doi:10.1111/sbr.12124.
[14] A. Al Saif, E. Waly, S. Alsenany, The prediction of falls among older people in Saudi Arabia, J. Am. Sci. 8 (6) (2012), 692–700.
[15] M. AbuRuz, et al., Quality of life for Saudi patients with heart failure: a cross-sectional correlational study, Glob. J. Health Sci. 8 (3) (2015) 49–58, doi:10.5539/gjhs.v8n3p49.
[16] M. Albugami, et al., Health care maintenance of Saudi elderly women in outpatient clinics, Am. J. Intern. Med. 3 (5) (2015) 197, doi:10.11648/j.ajim.20150305.11.
[17] J. McMurray, Concise Guide to the Management of Heart Failure, World Health Organization (1996), doi:10.1016/S1388-9842(00)00077-5. PMID: 11416373.
[18] M.A. Hossain, et al., A framework for a context-aware elderly entertainment support system, Sensors 14 (6) (2014) 10538–10561, doi:10.3390/s140610538.
[19] M. Alsulami, A. Atkins, R. Campion, An enhanced conceptual model for using ambient assisted living to provide a home proactive monitoring system for elderly Saudi Arabians, Proc. IEEE/ACS 14th International Conference on Computer Systems and Applications, (2017) 1443–1449.
[20] O. Grady, et al., Towards evolutionary ambient assisted living systems, J. Ambient Intell. Humaniz. Comput. *1* (1) (2010) 15–29.
[21] P. Rashidi, A. Mihailidis, A survey on ambient-assisted living tools for older adults, IEEE J. Biomed. Health Inf. 17 (3) (2013) 579–590, doi:10.1109/JBHI.2012.2234129.
[22] C. Jaschinski, S.Ben Allouch, An extended view on benefits and barriers of ambient assisted living solutions, Int. J. Adv. Life Sci. 7 (1) (2015) 40–53.
[23] C. Siegel, T.E. Dorner, Information technologies for active and assisted living—influences to the quality of life of an ageing society, Int. J. Med. Inform. 100 (2017) 32–45, doi:10.1016/j.ijmedinf.2017.01.012.
[24] M. Hersh, Overcoming barriers and increasing independence – service robots for elderly and disabled people, Int. J. Adv. Robot. Syst (2015), doi:10.5772/59230.
[25] N. Balta-Ozkan, et al., Social barriers to the adoption of Smart Homes, Energy Policy 63 (2013) 363–374, doi:10.1016/j.enpol.2013.08.043.

[26] L. Liu, et al., Smart Homes and home health monitoring technologies for older adults: a systematic review, Int. J. Med. Inf. 91 (2016) 44–59, doi:10.1016/j.ijmedinf.2016.04.007.
[27] A. Mageroski, et al., Impact of wireless communications technologies on elder people healthcare: Smart Home in Australia, In: Proc. 13th International Joint Conference on Computer Science and Software Engineering, JCSSE 2016, 2016, doi:10.1109/JCSSE.2016.7748862.
[28] B. Hafidh, et al., SITE: the simple internet of things enabler for Smart Homes, IEEE Access 5 (2017) 2034–2049, doi:10.1109/ACCESS.2017.2653079.
[29] X. Cai, et al., Infrared human posture recognition method for monitoring in Smart homes based on hidden Markov model, Sustainability 8 (9) (2016) 892, doi:10.3390/su8090892.
[30] C. Wilson, T. Hargreaves, R. Hauxwell-Baldwin, Benefits and risks of Smart home technologies, Energy Policy 103 (2017) 72–83, doi:10.1016/j.enpol.2016.12.047.
[31] E. Pardo, D. Espes, P. Le-Parc, A framework for anomaly diagnosis in Smart homes based on ontology, Procedia Comput. Sci 83 (Ant) (2016) 545–552, doi:10.1016/j.procs.2016.04.255.
[32] M.M. Baig, H. Gholamhosseini, M.J. Connolly, A comprehensive survey of wearable and wireless ECG monitoring systems for older adults, Med. Biol. Eng. Comput. 51 (2013) 485–495, doi:10.1007/s11517-012-1021-6.
[33] M. Chan, et al., Wearable systems : current status and future challenges, Artif. Intell. Med. 56 (2012) 137–156.
[34] A. Arshad, et al., A study on health monitoring system: recent advancement, IIUM Eng. J. 15 (2) (2014) 87–99.
[35] GfK (2015) Smart Home Making the Smart Home a Reality. https://cdn2.hubspot.net/hubfs/2405078/cms-pdfs/fileadmin/user_upload/dyna_content/global/documents/reports/gfk-smart-home-teaserdeck-global.pdf [Accessed: 4 November 2017].
[36] Km. Morris, et al., Smart-Home technologies to assist older people to live well at home, J. Aging Sci. 01 (01) (2013) 1–9, doi:10.4172/2329-8847.1000101.
[37] M. Alsulami, A. Atkins, Elderly Saudi Arabians' Perceptions and Attitudes Towards Using Ambient Assisted Living Technologies, Proc. 64 The IIER International Conference, 2016, doi:10.13140/RG.2.1.3170.5209.
[38] M. Alsulami, A. Atkins, Factors Influencing ageing population for adopting ambient assisted living technologies in the Kingdom of Saudi Arabia, Ageing Int. 41 (2016) 227–239, doi:10.1007/s12126-016-9246-6.
[39] United Nations, Department of Economic and Social Affairs, P. D. (2019) World Population Prospects 2019: Volume I: Comprehensive Tables, World Population Prospects 2019. http://www.ncbi.nlm.nih.gov/pubmed/12283219 [Accessed: 20 August 2020].
[40] The Chartered Institute of Building (2007) The Impact of the Ageing Population. https://www.ciob.org/sites/default/files/CIOB%20research%20-%20The%20Impact%20of%20the%20Ageing%20Population%20on%20the%20Construction%20Industry_0.pdf [Accessed 17 May 2016].
[41] United Nations (2013) World Population Ageing 2013 Report, Division, Department of Economic and Social Affairs Population. https://www.un.org/en/development/desa/population/publications/pdf/ageing/WorldPopulationAgeing2013.pdf [Accessed 5 May 2017].
[42] M.T. Yasamy, T. Dua, M. Harper, S. Saxena, (2013). Mental health of older adults, addressing a growing concern. World Health Organization. http://www.who.int/mental_health/world-mental-health-day/WHO_paper_wmhd_2013.pdf [Accessed 10 April 2016].
[43] United Nations, World Population Ageing, 2019 (2019) World Population Ageing 2019, Economic and Social Affairs, Population Division. http://link.springer.com/chapter/10.1007/978-94-007-5204-7_6 [Accessed 5 August 2020].

[44] T. Altamimi, Healthy aging conceptualizations in Saudi Arabia : a systematic review, Int. J. Med. Sci. Public Health 5 (04) (2016), doi:10.5455/ijmsph.2016.25122015349.
[45] Statistics, S. G. A. for (2019) Saudi Census. https://www.stats.gov.sa/ar/43 (Accessed: 26 August 2020).
[46] Saudi General Authority for Statistic (2017) 'Elderly Survey'. https://www.stats.gov.sa/sites/default/files/elderly_survey_2017en.pdf [Accessed 5 October 2017].
[47] J. M. Bauer, et al., Impacts of informal caregiving on caregiver employment, health and family, J. Popul. Ageing 8 (3) (2015) 113–145.
[48] World Health Organization (2015) World Report on Ageing and Health. http://apps.who.int/iris/bitstream/handle/10665/186463/9789240694811_eng.pdf;jsessionid=7CDED99798C66A56F0B78AA82EDABEAC?sequence=1 [Accessed 5 May 2017].
[49] Government Office for Science (2016) Future of an Ageing Population. https://assets.publishing.service.gov.uk/government/uploads/system/uploads/attachment_data/file/816458/future-of-an-ageing-population.pdf [Accessed 5 May 2017].
[50] W. He, D. Goodkind, P. Kowal, An Aging World : 2015 International Population Reports, U.S. Census Bureau, 2016. doi: P95/09-1. https://www.census.gov/content/dam/Census/library/publications/2016/demo/p95-16-1.pdf [Accessed 5 May 2017].
[51] Standard & Poor's Financial Services LLC (2016) Global Aging 2016: 58 Shades Of Gray. https://www.spglobal.com/en/research-insights/articles/global-aging-2016-58-shades-of-gray- [Accessed 5 May 2017].
[52] Public Pension Agency (2015) Annual Statistical Report-2015. https://www.stats.gov.sa/en/403 [Accessed 5 May 2017].
[53] N. Alazzam, Public pension agency in Saudi Arabia, Int. J. Sci. Eng. Res. 7 (3) (2016) 776–778.
[54] Strulik, H. and Werner, K. (2012) Life expectancy, labor supply, and long-run growth: reconciling theory and evidence. Center for European, Governance and Economic Development Research Discussion Papers 141, University of Goettingen, Department of Economics.
[55] Mckinsey Global Institute, Saudi Arabia Beyond Oil : The Investment and Productivity Transformation, Mckinsey Global Institute, Saudi Arabia, 2015.
[56] M. Almalki, G. Fitzgerald, M. Clark, Health care system in Saudi Arabia: an overview, East. Mediterr. Health J. 17 (10) (2011) 784–793, doi:10.1111/j.1466-7657.2011.00890.x.
[57] O. Safi, The challenges for Saudi Arabia health care system, Indian J. Appl. Res. 6 (2016) 231–233.
[58] Ministry of Health (2015) MOH-Statistical Book, Saudi Arabia. https://www.moh.gov.sa/en/Ministry/Statistics/book/Documents/StatisticalBook-1436.pdf [Accessed 5 May 2017].
[59] H.T.A. Khan, G.W. Leeson, H Findlay, Attitudes towards bearing the cost of care in later life across the world, Illn. Crisis Loss 21 (1) (2013) 49–69, doi:10.2190/IL.21.1.e.
[60] J. Parkash, M.Z. Younis, W. Ward, Healthcare for the ageing populations of countries of Middle East and North Africa, Ageing Int 40, (2015) 3–12, doi:10.1007/s12126-012-9150-7.
[61] Al-shabani, M. A. (2005) 'Active Ageing and Retiree Participation in the Kingdom of Saudi Arabia', (Ph.D. thesis), White Rose University Consortium, UK.
[62] Ministry of Health, Health Statistics Annual Book, Saudi Arabian Ministry of Health, 2013.
[63] A.H. Alanazi, Patients perception about home health care, J. Res. Method Educ. 4 (6) (2014) 40–47.
[64] ATKearney and Consumer Goods Forum, Understanding the Needs and Consequences of the Ageing Consumer, Consumer Goods Forum, 2013. https://www.theconsumergoodsforum.com/wp-content/uploads/2017/11/CGF-Understanding-the-Needs-of-ageing_consumer_report.pdf [Accessed 19 October 2016].

[65] Financial Conduct Authority (2016) Ageing Population and Financial Services. https://www.fca.org.uk/publication/discussion/dp16-01.pdf [Accessed 27 September 2018].

[66] Savills World Research (2015) Spotlight Housing an Ageing Population. https://www.savills.co.uk/research_articles/229130/193071-0 [Accessed 20 September 2018].

[67] Saudi General Authority for Statistic (2015) Statistical Yearbook 2015. https://www.stats.gov.sa/en/403 [Accessed 20 August 2018].

[68] Ministry of Foreign Affairs (2016) Ministry of Foreign Affairs. https://www.mofa.gov.sa/ [Accessed 20 August 2018].

[69] H. Almasabi, An overview of health system in Saudi Arabia, Res. J. Med. Sci. 7 (3) (2013) 70–74, doi:10.3923/rjmsci.2013.70.74.

[70] A.M. Alshahrani, S.A. Raheel, Health-care system and accessibility of dental services in Kingdom of Saudi Arabia : an update, J. Int. Oral Health 8 (2016) 883–887, doi:10.2047/jioh-08-08-10.

[71] M.A. Ismail, What derives public health expenditures in Saudi Arabia? Macro-econometric analysis, Int. J. Sci. Res. 4 (9) (2015) 623–629.

[72] Ministry of Finance (2019) 'Budget Statement Fiscal Year 2019'. https://www.mof.gov.sa/en/budget/2019/Documents/Budget%20Statement%202019.pdf [Accessed 8 August 2020].

[73] National Transformation Program (2016) National Transformation Program 2020. https://www.vision2030.gov.sa/v2030/vrps/ntp/ [Accessed 23 June 2021].

[74] Planning and Development Directorate (2016) Annual Statistics Book- Ministry of Labour and Social Development 2016. https://hrsd.gov.sa/sites/default/files/uploads/v.26%20%D8%A7%D9%84%D8%AA%D9%82%D8%B1%D9%8A%D8%B1%20%D8%A7%D9%84%D8%B3%D9%86%D9%88%D9%8A%202016.pdf [Accessed 23 June 2021].

[75] D. Crowder, Building a Web site For Dummies, John Wiley & Sons, NJ, 2010.

[76] I. Pires, et al., From data acquisition to data fusion: a comprehensive review and a roadmap for the identification of activities of daily living using mobile devices, Sensors 16 (2) (2016) 184, doi:10.3390/s16020184.

[77] L.Da Xu, et al., Internet of Things in industries : a survey, IEEE Trans. Ind. Inform. 10 (2014) 2233–2243, doi:10.1109/TII.2014.2300753.

[78] K. Srivastava, P.S.V.S. Sridhar, A Dehwal, Data integration challenges and solutions : a study, Int. J.Adv. Res. Comput. Sci. Softw. Engi. 2 (7) (2012) 34–37 doi: ISSN: 2277 128X.

[79] A. Alharthi, et al., An overview of cloud services adoption challenges in higher education institutions, Proc. 2nd International Workshop on Emerging Software as a Service and Analytics, 2015 102–109, doi:10.5220/0005529701020109.

[80] F. Alharbi, A. Atkins, C. Stanier, Understanding the determinants of cloud computing adoption in Saudi healthcare organisations, Complex Intell. Syst. 2 (2016) 155–171, doi:10.1007/s40747-016-0021-9.

[81] KPMG (2014) Cloud Economics: Making the Business Case for Cloud. https://assets.kpmg/content/dam/kpmg/pdf/2015/11/cloud-economics.pdf [Accessed 17 June 2017]

[82] I. Nonaka, R. Toyama, N. Konno, SECI, Ba and leadership : a unified model of dynamic knowledge creation, Long Range Planning 33 (2000) 5–34.

[83] K.P. Tripathi, A review on knowledge-based expert system : concept and architecture, Int. J. Comput. Appl. (Special issue on Artificial Intelligence Techniques - Novel Approaches & Practical Applications) 4 (4) (2011) 19–23, doi:10.5120/2845-226.

[84] S. Liao, Knowledge management technologies and applications—literature review from 1995 to 2002, Expert Syst. Appl. 25 (2) (2003) 155–164, doi:10.1016/S0957-4174(03)00043-5.

[85] I. Bichindaritz, et al., Integrating case-based reasoning, rule-based reasoning and intelligent information retrieval for medical problem-solving, Inf. Retr. (1998) 22–27.

[86] S.L. Syed-Abdullah, et al., Rule based reasoning and case based reasoning techniques for juvenile delinquency legal reasoning model, Proc. 5th International Conference on Computing and Informatics, ICOCI 2015, Istanbul, Turkey. Istanbul, 2015 677–683.
[87] A.A. AlYami, A.S. Atkins, R. Campion, Performance improvement in hospital management using RFID and ZigBee technologies for tracking and monitoring patients and assets in Saudi Arabia, Int. J. Manage. Appl. Sci. 2 (9) (2016) 66–69.
[88] S. Few, Information Dashboard Design; Displaying Data For At-A-Glance Monitoring, 2nd edn., Analytics Press, CA, USA, 2013.
[89] W. Noonpakdee, et al., A framework for analyzing and developing dashboard templates for small and medium enterprises, Proc. 5th International Conference on Industrial Engineering and Applications, ICIEA 2018, IEEE, 2018, pp. 479–483, doi:10.1109/IEA.2018.8387148.
[90] A. Sorour, et al., Integrated dashboards with social media analysis capabilities for monitoring quality in higher education institutions, Proc. 12th International Conference on Education and New Learning Technologies, 6-7 July, 2020 2862–2870.
[91] B. Scholtz, A. Calitz, R. Haupt, A business intelligence framework for sustainability information management in higher education, Int. J. Sustain. High. Educ. 19 (2) (2018) 266–290. https://doi.org/10.1108/IJSHE-06-2016-0118 Accessed 23 April 2018.
[92] Diffily, S. (2006) The Website Manager's Handbook. http://www.diffily.com/book/website_development.pdf [Accessed 23 June 2021].
[93] American Society on Aging (2020) American Society on Aging. https://www.asaging.org/ [Accessed 23 June 2021].
[94] Age UK (2020) Age UK. https://www.ageuk.org.uk/ [Accessed 23 June 2021].
[95] Aging in America (2020) 'Aging in America'. https://aginginamerica.org/ [Accessed 23 June 2021].
[96] EuroHealthNet (2020) EuroHealthNet Health Ageing. https://eurohealthnet.eu/phase/eurohealthnet%E2%80%99s-portal-healthy-ageing [Accessed 23 June 2021].
[97] My Ageing Parent (2017) My Ageing Parent. https://myageingparent.com/ [Accessed 23 June 2017].
[98] Nielsen, J. (1999) 10 Good Deeds in Web Design, Alertbox Website. http://www.arraydev.com/commerce/delibadmin/TenGoodDeeds.htm [Accessed 15 September 2017].
[99] Al-salebi, F. A. (2010) The Important Characteristics to Make a Good Website. Graduate Research Paper, Rochester Institute of Technology, USA.
[100] J. Nielsen, H. Loranger, Prioritizing Web Usability, Pearson Education, London, UK, 2006.
[101] Wix.com (2017) wix.com [Accessed 23 June 2017].
[102] S.M. Steele, Program evaluation- a broader definition, J. Ext. 8 (2) (1970) 5–17.
[103] J. Nielsen, Usability 101: Introduction to Usability, Nielsen Norman Group, CA, 2012.
[104] T. Issa, P. Isaias, Sustainable Design: HCI, Usability and Environmental Concerns, Springer, Cham, 2015, pp. i–iii, doi:10.1007/978-1-4471-6753-2.
[105] H. Layla, M. Anne, P. Steve, E-commerce websites for developing countries – a usability evaluation framework, Online Inform. Rev. J. 37 (2) (2013) 231–251, doi:10.1108/OIR-10-2011-0166 dx.doi.org/.
[106] L. Hasan, Evaluating the usability of educational websites based on students' preferences of design characteristics, Int. Arab J. e-Technol. 3 (3) (2014) 179–193.
[107] J. Nielsen, 10 Usability Heuristics for User Interface Design a, Nielsen Norman Group, CA, 1995.
[108] J. Nielsen, Severity ratings for usability problems, Papers and Essays, 54 (1995), 1–2.
[109] W. Bartels, M. Breeze, N. Peterson, Evaluating Web sites through the use of Focus Group, Center for Natural Resources (CNR), University of Florida, USA, 2003. https://ufdc.ufl.edu/IR00002482/00001 [Accessed 23 June 2021].
[110] Ministry of Health (2017). Statistical Year Book. Available from: stat@moh.gov.sa.

CHAPTER

4

Long-term nursing care at home: challenges and technology-driven solution approaches: the case of German healthcare system

Thierry Oscar

Department Of Drug Regulatory Affairs, RFW-University of Bonn, Germany

LEARNING OBJECTIVES

- This chapter has designed and implemented an Internet-of-Things-enabled home-based care system and living assistance conceptualizing Smart home automation multidimensionality. This is a great contribution and novelty, which combines nursing care and living assistance paradigm as a whole under the term home-based care.
- The proposed home-based care system goes beyond health, medical, and nursing care, and living assistance. It cares for the caregivers, especially for young carers in relieving them with the objectives to improve their quality-of-life and prevent them from mortgage their futures.
- This approach prevents patients and caregivers from social isolation, stress, depression, and burn-out.

4.1 Introduction

Care for older people is becoming challenging. High-income countries(HIC) are facing a nursing shortage crisis due to their fast-growing aging population. An increasing number of older people are requesting nursing care

Smart Home Technologies and Services for Geriatric Rehabilitation
DOI: https://doi.org/10.1016/B978-0-32-385173-2.00003-5

while the capacity of healthcare systems worldwide is decreasing due to practiced financial austerity policies, workforce shortage, hospital and/or nursing home beds occupied by people requesting less healthcare, etc.

Aging-in-place is the most practiced solutions to overcome the nursing shortage crisis. These approaches are widely supported and enabled by information and communication technology. Technology-enabled aging in place pursues the objective to keep older people in their common communities as long as possible and offer them independent living, and empower and prevent them from social isolation. Despite technological support, older people still need assistance to accomplish certain tasks. Prior studies have revealed that young and adult informal and family caregivers, caring for their close relatives at home, are facing high burdens. This chapter will focus on the German nursing care shortage crisis.

4.1.1 The world demographic

The population of HIC constituted a huge number of older and young people (aged ≥ 15 years). The older people in HIC belong to a rapid-growing group, while developing and low- and middle-income countries are bearing a high rate of young people with a median age of 15 years [1]. The median age in the HIC, especially in the European Union, was 36.5 years in 1995 and will be 47.6 years by 2060.

Cognitive impairments appear at an advanced age, but can also occur at a young age. Older people face age-related impairments such as Parkison diseases, Alzheimer's diseases, mental disorders/diseases, autonomy loss, dementia and cognitive impairments, hearing loss, etc. They, therefore, require intensive and effective nursing care. Most people aged 75+ years need round-the-clock nursing care [2].

4.1.2 Demography-related nursing care challenges

Skilled nurse shortage represents an unprecedented crisis in most HIC [3, 4]. Germany, an HIC, faces a nursing crisis that may be continuously accentuating due to the fast aging of its population. The number of people requiring nursing care will continuously increase. Therefore, the needs for the nursing workforce will subsequently increase. Antje, Jürgen, and Chrysanthi estimated that 130,000 more nursing staff will be needed in 2030 than in 2017 [5].

Owing to the nursing crisis in Germany, a workshop with theme: *"Nursing care at the border, Some preliminary remarks"* held in November 2016 in Mondorf-les-Bains, Luxembourg, had discussed different solutions approaches to mitigate the nursing crisis, for example, support the nursing care social aspect and encouraging the paradigm of ageing-in-place. The workshop participants have discussed ongoing social, demographic, economic changes and employment market constraints. It results from the meeting that the part of home-based nursing care is too low than that of ambulatory care for two major reasons: (1) Aging people mostly live alone and (2) financial issues [6].

Almost all age-related cognitive conditions are incurable and sometimes worsening, nursing care is concerned with relieving patients and improving their quality-of-life (QoL). However, the care needs of older people and people with chronic diseases go over and above nursing and medical care. These needs include daily living assistance in, for example, having social contact, going out, walking, visiting a doctor, doing physical activities, etc. Furthermore, older and patients with chronic diseases and/or mobility impairments aspire for living independently as possible.

4.1.3 Home nursing care and related concerns

Caring for a family member is challenging especially for working people and young family members.

There is empirical evidence that the burden of caring for an ill family member negatively impacts caregiver health. Caregivers especially those caring for a dementia patient are severely affected [7]. The literature review has revealed the negative impact of caring for a close relative on adult working life and young school performance. Many studies, for example [8], have pointed out the socioeconomic issues facing caregivers. People with dementia are subjected to forget to eat, drinking enough, and taking their medication, and request round-the-clock living assistance for common daily tasks such as opening windows.

4.1.3.1 Informal adult caregivers

Caring for a close relative implies high burdens on informal and family adult caregivers. Depending on whether the patient is rich or poor, caregivers have different feelings about the intensity of the burdens. The more the ill parent is rich the less the caregivers are feeling the burden because of the financial reward caregivers can expect. Many people are willing to care for their rich ill parent and thus share the burden. This is in line with one of the key findings of the study reported in [9], whereas the authors pointed out that the extent of the caring burden on a caregiver depends on the availability of another informal caregiver within the family. Table 4.1 summarizes an exhaustive literature review on burdens on adult caregivers in a home-based nursing care.

4.1.3.2 Informal young caregivers/carers

Young family members often care for their ill parents and perform various care-related activities [10]. However, this phenomenon is only poorly known to the general public [9]. Josef et al. have pointed out that 2%–8%

TABLE 4.1 Summary of health issues facing caregivers.

Pos.	Articles ***[title, authors(s), pub. year]***	**Burden on caregiver and health Issues faced**	**Digest/key findings/authors conclusions**
01	Dementia prevention, intervention, and care [7]	High burden on caregivers caring for dementia patients	• **Care for family carers** Family carers are at high risk of depression. Effective interventions, including STrAtegies for RelaTives (START) or Resources for Enhancing Alzheimer's Caregiver Health intervention (REACH), reduce the risk of depression, treat the symptoms, and should be made available. • **Technology** Technological interventions have the potential to improve care delivery but should not replace social contact.
02	Emerging roles for telemedicine and smart technologies in dementia care [22]	Increasing burden on family caregivers	• **Caregiver Burden** As the population with dementia expands and increases the burden on family caregivers, telemedicine and smart technologies have potential to support aging in place for PWD while reducing caregiver burden and its negative outcomes, improving quality of life for families experiencing dementia and reducing healthcare costs. • **Technology** Finally, the potential for technology to support dementia care at home may reduce healthcare expenditures secondary to formal care needs and premature institutional care. However, realizing the potential for technology to meet dementia care needs depends on several factors, including raising awareness of available technologies and their utility, promoting accessibility and affordability, and overcoming challenges to acceptance and use. • **Appeals/recommendation** Future research and continuous development are required to use advanced technology integrated with current dementia care.

03	Physical disability contributes to caregiver stress in dementia caregivers [28]	Caring for a dementia patient is stressful. Physical disabled and/or older caregivers are severely affected	• **Conclusion** Chronic disability as assessed by SF-12 PCS scores is independently associated with caregiver stress. These data suggest that caregivers of persons with dementia should be assessed for disabling physical conditions and mental health problems. Besides, reducing the impact of physical disability could ameliorate caregiver stress.
04	Dementia care: mental health effects, intervention strategies, and clinical implications [29]	Caregivers face eating disorders, high burden, distress	• **Abstract** Caring for elderly people with dementia is associated with well-documented increases in burden, distress, and decrements in mental health and wellbeing. More severe behavioural, cognitive, and functional impairments in a patient are associated with higher levels of burden and distress. Distress increases with care hours per week, number of tasks, and declining coping and support resources.
05	A systematic review of the prevalence and covariates of anxiety in caregivers of people with dementia [30]	High anxiety level on caregivers	• **Conclusions** Clinically significant anxiety affects about a quarter of CGs and is more common than in control populations.CG = Caregiver
06	Dementia behavioral and psychiatric symptoms: effect on caregiver's sleep [31]	Sleep disorder facing	• **Conclusions** Despite these limitations, this study adds to our body of knowledge regarding the complexity of problems that contribute to poor caregiver sleep. The present findings support previous findings that thePWD's nighttime behavior is a primary source of sleep disruption for many caregivers, but even nonresidential caregivers experience poor sleep. Besides, the present study provides new information about the relationship between the types and frequency of daytimeBPSDand caregivers' appraisal of their sleep quality. Caregivers reported poor sleep quality when they reported more frequent occurrences of nighttime disruptions by thePWD, more apathy, episodes of agitation, depression, or inappropriate behavior in thePWD.BPSD= behavioral and psychological symptoms of dementiaPWD's= persons with Alzheimer's and other dementias

(continued)

TABLE 4.1 (Cont'd)

Pos.	Articles *[title, authors(s), pub. year]*	Burden on caregiver and health Issues faced	Digest/key findings/authors conclusions
07	Factors determining the impact of caregiving on caregivers of elderly patients with dementia. A systematic literature review [32]	Depression	• **Results** Depression occurs in one in three caregivers and it occurs more frequently in those who care for patients with dementia than in caregivers of patients with other chronic illnesses.
08	The problem with "problem behaviors": a systematic review of the association between individual patient behavioral and psychological symptoms and caregiver depression and burden within the dementia patient-caregiver dyad [33]	Depression	• **Conclusion** The association between BPSDs and caregiverdepression and burden is proven
09	Caregiver burden for informal caregivers of patients with dementia: A systematic review [34]	Burden on caregivers	• **Conclusion** The study has identified the factors impacting caregiver burdens as following: 1. Caregiver sociodemographical factors, 2. Psychological factors and 3. Caregiving-related factors 4. The age of the caregiver and 5. The relationship with the patient

10	Correlates of Physical Health of Informal Caregivers: A Meta-Analysis [8]	Face financial and socialization issues (poor socioeconomic status)	• **Conclusion** The study concludes the following: • First, caregiving-related stressors affect caregivers' physical health, but these associations are weaker than the effects of stress on psychological health. • Second, feeling depressed is more strongly associated with caregivers' physical health than the absolute levels of caregiving demands. • Third, higher caregiving demands have a stronger impact on the physical health of older caregivers, dementia caregivers, and men, thus suggesting that these are additional risk factors for practitioners to be aware of.
11	Effectiveness of an Internet Intervention for Family Caregivers of People with dementia: Results of a Randomized Controlled Trial [35]	Psychological distress, depression, and anxiety	• **Conclusion** This study figured out that information on Dementia provided via the Internet with family caregivers can contribute to reducing care-related depression and anxiety.

of youths are caring for their parents [2]. Data collected in Africa and Asia indicate that this is a global phenomenon. Järkestig-Berggren et al. investigated the extent of the phenomenon of "young caregivers" in Sweden [11]. They found out that even young people aged 10 years are concerned. The study highlighted serious problems experienced by these children, such as psychological well-being problems, hyperactivity, and social problems.

Sharmila Parks wrote in a forum [[12]: *However young carers are at risk of social isolation and bullying, under-achievement, absenteeism from school, and physical and mental ill-health.*

Leu et al. also conducted a similar study [9] in Switzerland as Järkestig-Berggren et al. did in Sweden. They investigated many aspects of the "young carers" phenomenon and found out that certain young people, additionally, work outside to financially assist/help their family whose revenue decrease due to health problems.

Young caregivers face a high burden in terms of sibling care, domestic tasks, and caring activities. They experience bad school performance, or school abandonment, and suffer from mental disorders. Table 4.2 presents burdens on and challenges facing young caregivers/carers in a home-based care environment.

4.1.4 Family caregivers and older people's QoL

The older people's QoL in nursing homes has been well investigated. However, the QoL of people aging in place is more or less not investigated. Førsund et al. pointed out that the health-related QoL of dementia patients, living in a nursing home, could be impacted by structural and organizational characteristics of the home [13]. The authors have listed parameters such as room temperature, lighting, noise tolerance, convenable space, and the possibility of social, cognitive, and physical activities as a set of metrics to measure the QoL. To author's best knowledge, the impact of home-based nursing care on health-related QoL is not yet investigated.

Tables 4.3 and 4.4 define, respectively, QoL metrics/key performance indicator to assess and measure older people's *health* outcome-related QoL (HQoL) and intensity of burden on caregivers in home care.

4.1.5 Home nursing care technologies

Khosla et al.reported the use of assistive robots in home-based care to help older people [14]. Pieces of evidence have shown that assistive robots can assist older people to get socialized. Socialization could positively impact people's QoL. Sharif et al. proposed a telehealth system that makes people in home-based care or care-homes more independent and enables them an easy life [15].

TABLE 4.2 Summary of health issues facing young carers.

Pos.	Articles [title, authors(s), pub. year]	Caregiver burden and health issues faced	Digest/key findings/authors conclusions
01	Young Carers Research, Practice and Policy: An Overview and Critical Perspective on Possible Future Directions [2]	• No-training, no-paid carers face various risk such as developing infectious diseases • Experience various economic and social disadvantages • Bad school performance • Restrictive employment • Health and wellbeing issues • Social isolation	• **Conclusion** This work conducted a large-scale study on the topic and figured out the challenges and issues facing young carers caring for their parents
02	Children with ill parents: extent and nature of caring activities [10]	High extent of caring activities and domestic tasks	• **Conclusion** This study raises an important aspect of young carers' activities. It investigates factors associated with nature and the extent of caring activitiesThis study found that female children are more involved in the care of their parents. Children additionally perform domestic tasks, household management, financial/practical management, personal-, emotional-, and sibling care.
03	Young carers and young adult carers in Switzerland: Caring roles, ways into care and the meaning of communication [9]	Domestic tasks Caring activities Find the right information about caring for is challenging Young carers are vulnerable	• **An important key finding** The tasks, that young carers and young adult carers in Switzerland are responsible for depend on the nature of the illness or impairment of the person receiving care and the availability of other carers within the family. The intensity of the caring role varies from part-time to full-time responsibility

(continued)

TABLE 4.2 (Cont'd)

Pos.	Articles [title, authors(s), pub. year]	Caregiver burden and health issues faced	Digest/key findings/authors conclusions
04	A cross-sectional study on experiences of young adult carers compared to young adult noncarers: parentification, coping and resilience [36]	Face additional household and administrative burden	-
05	Young carers in Sweden: A pilot study of care activities, view of caring, and psychological well-being [11]	High burden including: • Personal care • Sibling care • Domestic tasks • Emotional care • Household management • Financial/practical	• **Key finding** Report a higher degree of negative consequences and lower psychological wellbeing than young carers in other countries.

TABLE 4.3 Older people's quality-of-life measurement metrics.

Metrics
Food and water intake level
Medication adherence level
Living comfort
Accident rate
Rate, intensity, and frequency of performing physical activities
Socialization level
Capacity, convenient, and frequency to go groceries
Capacity and frequency rate to visit a medical doctor

TABLE 4.4 Caregiver's quality-of-life measurement metrics.

Metrics
Intensity of care related daily tasks
Daily time volume for caring
Level of risk for burnout
Level of the care-related stress
Quality of work-care-life balance
Young caregivers' school performance
Adult caregivers' working performance level
Socialization level

Marikyan et al. reviewed Smart home automation applications and found that most Smart home automation application designs have led to partial or unidimensional services and user segments [16]. Only one paper has given insight into the paradigm and concept of the multidimensionality of Smart home automation [16].

Common ambient assistive living (AAL)/Smart home automation systems are unidimensional and only cover one aspect of home-based care. Additionally, most home automation systems intended to support the home-based care paradigm are also limited because they are unidimensional too.

Albahri et al. found that integrating telemedicine technology in network-enabled digital technologies presents certain advantages such as connecting healthcare machines to support home-based care systems [17], remotely monitor older people at home (telemonitoring), remote consultation (teleconsultation, telediagnostics), etc. Singh et al. designed an Internet-of-Things (IoT) based Smart home solution [18].

- *Smart home automation common definition*

A *Smart home* is a family home and/or building that incorporates modern automation systems (Table 4.5) and features a communication network that connects different house appliances to a central computer (locally or in the cloud) and enables remote control, monitoring, and access.

The most common Smart home automation systems are unidimensional or unifunctional; for example, they provide among others functions such as lighting control (energy management), temperature regulation (heater and air conditioning), multimedia devices management, as well as security and safety management such as monitoring and remote operating windows and doors.

TABLE 4.5 Multidimensional Smart home automation and Internet of things devices.

Device categories	**Devices**
Access monitoring	Smart garage doors Smart door locks Smart window locks
Incident management	Smart smoke detector
Energy and lighting	Smart plugs/outlets Smart temperature sensors Home energy monitors Smart thermostats Wireless Smart vents
Medical devices	Medical data gathering and health monitoring ECG Glucometer Thermometer Video camera (monitoring) Accelerometer Pulse oximeter Blood pressure monitor
Other devices	Home appliances Microwaves Fridge Television Furnace/kitchen Food and water intake Smart fridge Smart microwaves

• *Multidimensional concept of Smart home automation*
In contrary to unidimensional Smart home automation, multidimensional Smart home automation features a set of services from energy management to windows and doors management.
The multidimensional Smart home is customized to the user's needs in terms of services the user needs to manage all aspects of his everyday life.

4.1.5.1 *Overcoming the home nursing care issues and challenges*

Questions to be Answered by designing a technology-supported home-care system are as follows:

1. *Can technology empower people aging in place?*
Older people aging in place need, beyond the nursing care, daily living assistance. Providing living assistance to an ill person implies the 24-h presence of a third person (e.g., a family member) at his side. It will be difficult for one individual to assume such tasks. The caregivers, otherwise, will face various issues such as social isolation, joblessness, and financial issues.
2. *Can technology assist to reduce the intensity of burdens on caregivers in Homecare?*
A caregiver cannot alone provide 24-h nursing care to an ill parent. This challenge can only be tackled if all family members share the tasks or are assisted by external professional caregivers or technologies such as Smart home automation.
Many previous works carried out have shown the potentiality of Smart home automation supporting home-based healthcare.

4.2 Understanding the nursing shortage and long-term care at home

To understand why only a few older people age in their common communities, a survey was conducted.

The Snowball sampling approach is a suitable tool regarding the difficulties to easily sample older people. Collecting data in nursing homes is restrictive for medical and data privacy reasons as well as the distrust on the part of the elder. For these precise reasons, it was difficult to directly contact the participants. Participants have been therefore recruited and selected through insiders (care staff, family members, friends, etc.) for a cross-sectorial study.

Quantitative and qualitative data collection approach: Closed-ended and open-ended questions were used to collect quantitative and qualitative data. Older people living in nursing homes and their communities were interviewed about: (1) aging in place, (2) QoL in a nursing care home or at home, (3) needs and preferences, (4) nursing care crises and provided solutions, (5) the trend of aging in place, (6) challenges and issues facing home care, (7) the tendency to care for an ill person at home, etc.

Difficulty to collect data: It was difficult to include most nursing homes in the study because of data privacy and medical reasons. Furthermore, involved nursing care homes should have full anonymity to protect their business and resident data. Nurses with poor German knowledge were not allowed to participate in the interview. To overcome such obstacles, it is advised to elaborate multilingual questionnaires to assist non-German speaking people. To increase the nursing care homes' participation, a confidentiality clause needs to be concluded. The study outcomes can also be shared with the nursing care homes.

The technological aspect of the nursing care shortage is poorly handled in the literature. To collect enough information on the role of technology in mitigating the nursing shortage, interviews were conducted, and analysis of existing AAL system for example *Dorfgemeinschaft 2.0, Fürstenhof Projekt* in Germany, was carried out.

4.2.1 Older people in nursing care homes

Nursing homes are often in the headlines because of the inhuman conditions that the older people are subjected to, even though they are supposed to experience an improved QoL there. Below quotes from two online German newspapers present the conditions in some nursing care homes.

> *Neglected, depressed residents and exhausted, tired staff; inhumane conditions have long been the norm in nursing care* homes *[19].*

> *She told BR that the nurses had neglected her mother after an operation. She had vomited blood several times, but the nurse had only changed her clothes. Only at the daughter's request was an emergency doctor called. Other relatives reported that the toilet seats were dirty with excrement and that there was not enough food [20].*

The high nurse:patient ratio in terms of intensive burden on the nursing staff is the principal cause of these inhuman conditions that the older people are undergoing in some nursing care homes.

4.2.2 Nursing homes versus aging in place: older people preferences

Older people have shown a significant preference for "aging in place" and be independent as long as possible. Older people who prefer aging in place are those with good family support/community assistance (living together with or have good contact with children, grandchildren), and have good social contacts. Poor people, people with poor family support/community assistance feel comfortable at the nursing home. A total of 89% of people with poor familial support prefer aging in a residential nursing house, whereas 91% with good family support/community assistance prefer aging in place.

4.2.3 Caring for close relatives

A convenience sample (397 people) was interviewed on their preference to care for an ill family member, 233 (58.69%) reported preferring to care for the ill parent. They indicate the crisis as well as issues at some nursing homes are the main reasons for this preference. A total of 97(24.43%) prefer to send the ill parent to a nursing home because they are working and lack time to care for parent. Additionally, they indicated that the ill parent is safer at a nursing home than at home regarding the community environment. A total of 67 responders (16.87%) prefer to send their ill parents to a nursing home abroad for financial reasons.

Of 17 young carers interviewed, 15 (88.29%) are suffering from a mental disorder (stress, depression), 6 (35.29%) have abandoned the school while 10 (58.82%) experience bad school performance.

4.2.4 Aging in place supporting systems

1. *Smart homes projects*

   Chan et al. presented many Smart home projects, for example. ACHE in the United States, Welfare Techno-Houses in Japan (Asia), and Gloucester's Smart House under others in Europe. TERVA project in Finland only monitors the medical signal of patients lying at home. PROSAFE and ENABLE also focus on collecting and monitoring medical and biosignals. These projects and systems are unidimensional.
2. *IoT on Smart home system*

   Singh et al. carried out a study on the design of an IoT-enabled Smart home automation (IoTSHS) [18]. However, the solution that the authors proposed cannot be controlled remotely.

   Nayyar et al. present the "*BioSenHealth 1.0*" a novel Internet of Medical Things to remotely monitor patients and was tested in 50+ care units [21]. Such a system presents many advantages for caregivers who work outside and additionally have to care for an ill family member. They can remotely control many things around the patient, for example, assist him with medication and food intake. This kind of system can contribute to ensuring that the patient's adherence to the treatment as requested.

   A caregiver can interact remotely with an elderly adult using smartphones or PC cameras. Seniors suffering from anxiety or dementia can be reassured by seeing or interacting with their caregivers via video.

3. *Emerging roles for telemedicine and smart technologies in dementia care*
Bossen et al., in the conclusion of the study, stated that Smart home automation technology has shown promise to assist older people living in their common communities [22].

4.3 A Smart home automation technology-supported home care

The proposed approach aims at (1) providing living assistance to patients and empowering them, (2) contributing to lessening the burden on informal caregivers, especially the young carers, (3) preventing patients as well as the carer from social isolation, and (4) collecting patient-centric data for personalized treatment and for short response time in the case of emergency.

4.3.1 System requirements

The system should feature a patient-centric data perception unit so that authorized entities such as nursing care staff and patient relatives can ubiquitously process the stored data.

The *biosignals* have to be collected round the clock depending on the patient's health condition, and regardless of the location, indoor or outdoor, of the patient.

Behavioral data: Body expressions, behaviors, mimic, any physical activities should unobtructively[1] be recorded using a network capable video-camera, which will store the collected data in the local and remote servers.

Environmental data: In previous work, the authors have used a sensor network to collect indoor environmental data such as room temperature, the quantity of CO_2, and the indoor air quality. This construction needs to be included in the Smart home on IoT to collect data that can negatively impact patient health. An additional obtructive video chain should be installed in the entire living area.

Prediction and prevention: A machine learning processor, located in the cloud, should use these collected data for training purposes on one hand, and on the other hand for predicting patient behaviors, level of empowerment, expectations, physiological demands (such as thirst, hunger, go to the toilet, etc.) and cognitive decline [23, 24].

Food and water intake management: A system capable to autonomously and automatically order food and water should be provided. A "water and food dispenser (WaFoD)" should consist of a smart fridge, smart

[1]To prevent the older people from anxiety [24].

microwaves, and smart water dispenser. This system would enable and monitor food and water intake. The involved devices should be networking enable to connect to the IoT network.

4.3.2 System features

Based on the system requirements, system features the following.

4.3.2.1 *Prevent hunger and thirst*

A water and food dispensation and intake monitoring system is provided. It assists to prevent older people from hunger and thirst.

4.3.2.2 *Autonomous and automatic food and beverage order*

1. Present day's meal menu list;
2. The patient selects a menu or three (03) menus from his favorites based on historical data. A machine-learning algorithm could select a menu based on the day time, season, weather, etc.;
3. The selected food automatically ordered at a registered restaurant; and
4. Food is delivered.

4.3.2.3 *WaFoD (water and food dispensing)*

1. A special smart box is used to keep food.
2. The food is warm at appropriate times of the day like lunch or dinner time
3. The food then is served.

At each stage patients with cognitive impairment are guided through the different steps, for example, tell him to sit and eat at the table.

- *Reminder for family members:* WaFoD can also remind a family member to order food and drinks for the patient.

4.3.2.4 *Medication intake monitoring*

A drug box is a box with an integrated high-resolution camera, logs, any drug intake. The box features are planned to be extended with an automatic anomalies detector and recorder.

The caregivers can visualize the drug intake film in real time and can thus act accordingly.

4.3.2.5 *Indoor and outdoor physical exercises*

Recorded physical exercise films are displayed at scheduled times. The patient can then watch the film and train himself accordingly. To prevent the patient from falling and determine his position in real time, a network of biosensors called body area networking (BAN) and including accelerometer continually monitors the patient.

Any physical activities the patient performs are recorded.

4.3.2.6 *Monitor and control room ambient temperature*

This work will integrate the existing concept of room ambient temperature control and management that is well-established in the Smart home domain.

Noise and lighting control as well as incident management: This feature controls and manages noise and energy.

4.3.2.7 *Control windows and doors*

Doors and windows are continuously monitored. The system automatically closes in the case of high noise, rain, cold, etc., as well as at certain hours of the day.

4.3.2.8 *Daily living assistance and reminder*

A smartphone-based application and a reminder assist the patient in doing his daily tasks such as visiting a doctor, go to the grocery as long as he can do this. Data from the patient calendar are autonomously used to plan the day for the patient.

An Integrated Google navigation system is used to assist the patient to go out and come back without getting lost along the way. For dementia patients, indoor navigation is provided to guide them from one room to the next right room.

Living assistance for blind and deaf patients: Blind and deaf can benefit from indoor navigation too as well from the recent technology advancement such as the *Dot Braille Smartwatch* [https://www.dotincorp.com/] for blind people.

The living assistance functionality for the blind and deaf is not yet integrated or implemented. Though, many related works have been already done. This functionality can be based on existing systems such as that described in Guerrero et al. [25], where the authors have implemented an indoor navigation system for visually impaired people.

System data and data management: The following types of data are collected at regular intervals by the proposed multidimensional Smart home automation system by using corresponding hardware.

4.3.2.8.1 Room quality data

1. *Room temperature*: A comfortable ambient temperature is necessary for the mood elevation of older patients.
2. *Ambient air and air quality*: These refer to the condition or quality of air surrounding the patient in the outdoor/indoors.

4.3.2.8.2 Food and water intake data

The data about the participant's food and water intake are recorded.

4.3.2.8.3 Medical data

A variety of medical data are collected periodically using personal health devices and applications available in the market. The types of collected data are as follows:

4.3.2.8.3.1 Biosignals

1. *ECG* records the heart's rhythm and activity in the form of a line on a screen.
2. *Blood glucose level*: This parameter refers to the concentration of glucose present in the blood.
3. *Body temperature*: Body temperature is a measure of the body's ability to generate and get rid of heat.
4. *Blood pressure*: Blood pressure is a measure of the force of circulating blood on the walls of the arteries. Systolic blood pressure is measured when the heart beats while diastolic blood pressure is measured between heartbeats.
5. *Oxygen saturation*: Oxygen saturation is the fraction of oxygen-saturated hemoglobin relative to total hemoglobin in the blood.

4.3.2.8.3.2 Medication

1. *Adherence* (*time*): Medication adherence measures the extent to which patients take medication as prescribed by their doctors.

4.3.2.8.4 Others

1. *Fall and risks*: This parameter counts the number of falls experienced by a patient and stratification of fall risks.
2. *Indoor and outdoor physical activities*: Physical activities such as walking, cycling, climbing the stairs are measured.
3. *Appointment (with the medical doctor):* The prescribed schedule of appointments with the doctor and the appointments followed are kept track.

4.3.3 Architecture

The architecture of the proposed multidimensional system for home-based care and living assistance consists of the following four layers:

1. *Things layer*

   The network's things layer consists of Smart home and medical devices, which are shown in Figs. 4.1 and 4.2, respectively. Various data such as patient biosignals, room ambient temperature, physical exercises, food and water intake, and treatment adherence are collected at this stage through consumer devices equipped with a variety of sensors.

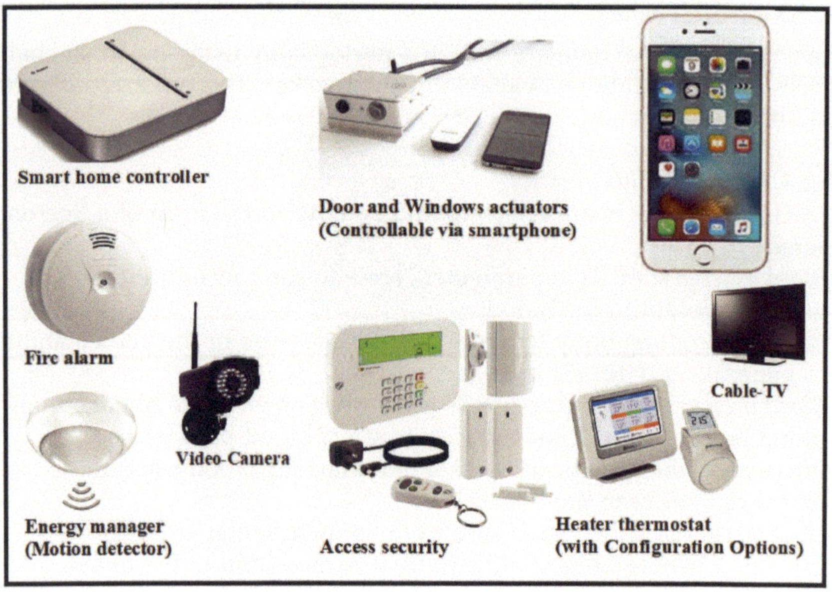

FIG. 4.1 Example of smart home automation equipments.

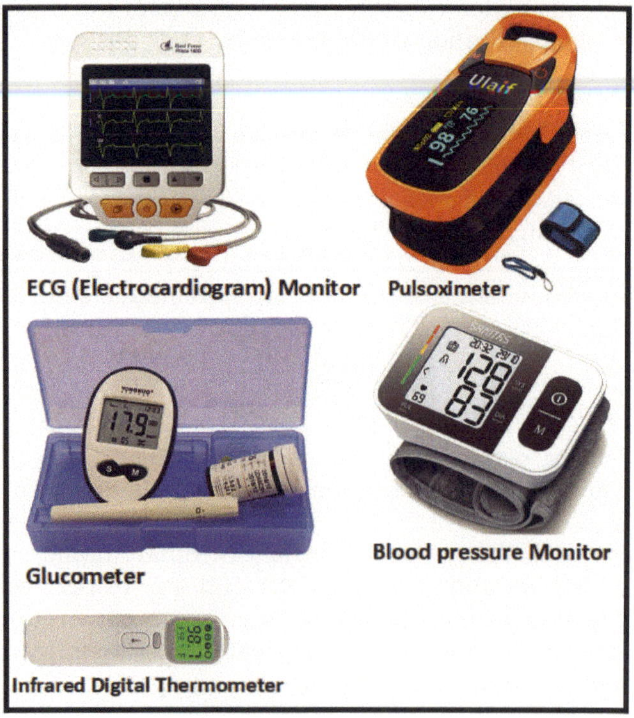

FIG. 4.2 Example of medical self-management devices.

2. *Edge layer*
The edge layer is based on the principles of edge computing and performs data processing closer to the source. The proximity of the processing unit with the data source removes processing latency. This allows large amounts of data to be processed near the source itself, resulting in a reduction of Internet bandwidth, lower costs, and applications that could be run within the boundary of the home without requiring Internet connectivity. The data processed at this stage are also forwarded to the cloud.
3. *Data aggregation/ingestion layer*
The data collected from individual devices are forwarded to the data aggregation layer. The devices at this layer are mainly smartphones that interface with multiple health devices and the Smart home hub that interfaces with multiple Smart-home devices. The devices at the data aggregation layer control and command individual devices at the network of things layer. Collected data are processed and prestored. For example, a mobile health app stores data related to the patient's all biosignals such as ECG, blood pressure, body temperature.
4. *Application and/or cloud layer*
The cloud layer stores data originating from multiple homes. These data are made available for further analysis that will help to improve the quality of health-care of patients. In our implementation, we used Amazon cloud services for the storage of data obtained from lower layers.

4.3.4 Concept

The system provides the following novel features beyond the classic Smart home automation features such as energy saving, incident monitoring, smoke monitoring, room-temperature management: (1) a medical data collection unit, (2) water drink, food intake, and treatment adhesions management unit, and (3) outdoor and indoor activities management unit.

4.3.4.1 *Data perception*

Medical data

Biosignals: Actually, medical treatments are based on narrative data provided by the patient (called patient-centered). Data emanating from a patient could be subjective, incomplete, or intentionally biased. To perform an accurate diagnosis, complementary medical exams are, therefore, often necessary. Precisely for these reasons, autonomously gathering patient biosignals, using modern technology such as the IoT to autonomously and automatically collect patient biosignals, is mandatory. Such data are called patient-centric and are complete. Patient-centric data give a detailed tableau of the patient's health state.

- *Patient-centered data versus patient-centric data*

  Patient-centered data are narrative data emanated from the patient or his relative. Particularly, the information provided by older people can be biased and/or incomplete because older people are cognitively impaired and are thus forgetful. *Patient-centric data* are gathered using (modern) information technology systems such as wireless sensors networks, the IoT, or BAN, which connects the patient to the IoT system. Collected data are preprocessed near the things (edge computing) and sent to the local server through the IoT-Gateway using MQTT (message queuing telemetry transport) broker according to data transfer protocol. IoT-based medical monitoring systems present various benefits for the patient and caregivers. Patient-centric data can support personalized care.
- *Data security (privacy, protection)*

  Data must be encrypted during an exchange. The HL7 format could be adopted to prevent from interoperability issues. Further HL7/FHIR with blockchain security technology could be used to exchange data

  Environmental data

  Ambient data need to be collected to analyze the quality of the air surronding the older people.

4.3.5 Design

4.3.5.1 Building WaFoD

The smart fridge is combined with the smart microwave and the water dispenser. Food stored in the fridge can autonomously move from the fridge to the microwave oven and get warmed. The Smart home automation controller manages the entire system. Patient family members can remotely control the WaFoD. The WaFoD can alert family members if the patient does not take his food or does not drink water served by the system. Though, one question that arises is: how a patient with mobility impairment can be served?

Assistive robots in older healthcare are well-achieved today [26, 27]. So it will be judicious to add an assistive robot to the WaFoD system, which will assist the mobility impaired patient in the absence of the caregiver.

WaFoD system should be designed as a cloud-based IoT platform, whose stack layers are: (1) Data perception unit(s) or the things consist of the smart fridge, the smart microwave, and the smart water dispenser, (2) the IoT-gateway located on a local copy of the remote server on the cloud. The IoT gateway connects the WaFoD to the cloud throughout the Smart home controller and enables data preprocessing in the near of the edge (edge computing), (3) IoT-core features consist of infrastructure, communication, data collection, etc., (4) the applications run on the cloud and perform complex and memory consuming computing tasks such as order food and water, predict patient food and beverage preferences (machine learning based application), etc.

4.3.5.2 WaFoD features

WaFoD features are (1) a reminder alarm that regularly requests the patient to drink water, (2) automatically dispenses beverage (hot drinks, soft drinks, water) according to a machine learning algorithm. The algorithm takes into account parameters such as time, weather, day time, room temperature, etc., (3) a logger: water and food intake protocol, (4) an emergency alert system that can autonomously alert the healthcare professionals, (5) display menu pictures through the TV. The food menu is sent by the restaurant to the WaFoD system via the cloud.

4.3.5.3 Medication adherence management

Like WaFoD, the medication adherence management system is also a cloud-based IoT platform. A medicine box equipped with sensors should be provided to assist the patient to adhere to the treatment. The box should register any medicine intake. As a reminder, the medicine box assists the patient in adhering to the medication. It alerts the carer in case the patient does not take his medicine on time or at all. Furthermore, the box should keep the medicine at an appropriate temperature.

The box is connected to the IoT Gateway and uses RFID technology to detect if the patient takes the medicine. A medical health record application in the cloud records and processes data about medication adherence. To assure that the patient takes the medicine a video camera should be provided to monitor the drug intake.

The architecture of the medication adherence system is similar to WaFoD's. The things are: (1) sponsored medicine box, (2) video camera for medication monitoring.

4.3.5.4 Indoor activities

Indoor activities consist of doing physical activités, watching TV, walking in the room, etc. A touchscreen TV that can display some information at there scheduled time is connected to a server.

The connected multimedia devices such as TV would display physical exercises to assist the patient to have some physical exercise. The patient can follow the moves and perform physical activities.

4.3.5.5 Outdoor activities

Older people tend to be socially isolated. This fact impacts their behaviors. Many older people visit a doctor only because they are looking for social contacts.

To prevent older people from social isolation, outdoor navigation based on Google Navigation should be provided. The main objectives of this solution are to guide older people when they are outside and empower them. Enabling the older to participate in outdoor activity will prevent them from social isolation. Similarly, it can be done for medical visits

4.3.6 System hardware

These hardware devices only need to be installed and connected to corresponding applications using Internet connectivity.

4.3.6.1 Feature extension

The work reported in this chapter has explored the trends of "aging in place," challenges and issues faced by young as well as an informal carer in home-based nursing care. The main objectives of this study were to assist young and informal carers in their daily tasks, improve their QoL, and prevent them from social isolation. Particularly, young carers would be assisted and prevented from mortgaging their futures.

Many research works have been carried out in the field of Smart homes and independent living and well "aging in place." Aging in place becomes more comfortable and smarter for the older. However, these said works have failed to provide a global Smart home automation solution (*multidimensional as well as multifunctional Smart home automation*) that takes into account the carer as well as the patient's perspectives and needs.

The study reported in this chapter has analyzed the challenges and issues facing home-based care from both patient's and caregiver's perspectives and proposed an appropriate solution approach that shows promise to lessen the high burden on the carers and provides, beyond the medical consideration, daily living assistance to the patients.

Future works: The upcoming works should aim at designing and implementing a human hologram for assisting people in home-based care. A human hologram can simulate a family member and give instructions or discuss it with the patient at home.

1. *Virtual human presence (hologram)*

The results of the present chapter have demonstrated a great impact of the presence of a family member on the patient's health outcomes and his HQoL.

Preventing from isolation by using hologram during the absence of family members or caregivers will, therefore, be investigated and implemented.

2. *Wearable for older people feeling*

Many prior studies have well achieved remote room-temperature settings and regulation. However, one can feel hot or cold regardless of the room temperature due to medicine intake or after-physical exercises. Temperature feelings can relate to the treatment one is undergoing. Though, to best of author's knowledge, there is no system to automatically and autonomously determine the appropriate temperature for the patient. We, therefore, project a wearable solution able to verify what the patient in terms of temperature is feeling and thus regulate the heater appropriately.

3. *Assisting blind and deaf people and indoor navigation*

The present proposed system faces some limitations. Deaf and blind people cannot adequately be assisted as appropriate devices are missing. The forthcoming work would therefore also focus on working out on approaches to help this category of patients.

4. *Assistive robot for WaFoD*

To lessen the burden on caregivers, an assistive robot is planned to be launched in the WaFoD system to assist the patient to take food and drink. The robot can play additional roles. As the WaFoD was simulated in the scope of this study, it is planned to build the WaFoD as a Smart home solution for aging in place. Discussions are being conducted with the industry.

References

[1] United Nations, Department of Economics and Social Affairs PD. World population prospects: The 2017 Revision [Internet]. Vol. II, Demographic Profiles (ST/ESA/SER.A/400). 2017. http://www.ncbi.nlm.nih.gov/pubmed/12283219 (Accessed 23 June 2021).

[2] S. Joseph, J. Sempik, A. Leu, S. BeckerYoung Carers Research, Practice and policy: an overview and critical perspective on possible future directions, Adolesc. Res. Rev 0123456789 (5) (2020) 77–99. doi: https://doi.org/10.1007/s40894-019-00119-9.

[3] X. Zhang, D. Tai, H. Pforsich, V.W. Lin, United States registered nurse workforce report card and shortage forecast: a revisit, Am. J. Med. Qual 33 (3) (2018) 229–236.

[4] M.S. Weaver, B. Wichman, S. Bace, D. Schroeder, C. Vail, C. Wichman, et al., Measuring the impact of the home health nursing shortage on family caregivers of children receiving palliative care, J. Hosp. Palliat. Nurs 20 (3) (2018) 260–265.

[5] A. Schwinger, J. Klauber, C. Tsiasioti, Pflegepersonal heute und morgen, in: K. Jacobs, A. Kuhlmey, S. Greß, J. Klauber, A. Schwinger (Eds.), Pflege-Report 2019, Springer Berlin Heidelberg, Berlin, Heidelberg, 2020, pp. 3–21. https://doi.org/10.1007/978-3-662-58935-9. (Accessed 23 June 2021).

[6] M. Breinbauer, R. Jacob, N. Richter, J. Kopp, Häusliche Pflege in der Region Trier, in: R Münnich, J Kopp (Eds.), Pflege an Der Grenze, Wiesbaden: Springer Fachmedien, Wiesbaden, 2019, pp. 149–177. https://doi.org/10.1007/978-3-658-19575-5_7.

[7] G. Livingston, A. Sommerlad, V. Orgeta, S.G. Costafreda, J. Huntley, D. Ames, et al., Dementia. prevention,. intervention,. and. care, Lancet 390 (10113) (2017) 2673–2734, doi:10.1016/S0140-6736(17)31363-6.

[8] M. Pinquart, S. Sörensen, Correlates of physical health of informal caregivers: a meta-analysis sociodemographic variables, J. Gerontol. Psychol. Sci. 62 (2) (2007) 126–137, doi: https://doi.org/10.1093/geronb/62.2.P126, http://psychsocgerontology.oxfordjournals.org/.

[9] A. Leu, M. Frech, C. Jung, Young carers and young adult carers in Switzerland: caring roles, ways into care and the meaning of communication, Heal. Soc. Care. Community 26 (6) (2018) 925–934.

[10] E.K. Kallander, B.M. Weimand, S. Becker, B. Van Roy, K. Hanssen-Bauer, K. Stavnes, et al., Children with ill parents: extent and nature of caring activities, Scand. J. Caring Sci 32 (2) (2018) 793–804.

[11] U. Järkestig-Berggren, A.S. Bergman, M. Eriksson, G. Priebe, Young carers in Sweden—A pilot study of care activities, view of caring, and psychological well-being, Child. Fam. Soc. Work 24 (2) (2019) 292–300.

[12] RE: Young Carers Br. J. of Gen. Pract. 2014. https://bjgp.org/content/re-young-carers (Accessed 4 June 2019).

[13] L.H. Førsund, E.K. Grov, A.S. Helvik, L.K. Juvet, K. Skovdahl, S. Eriksen, The experience of lived space in persons with dementia: a systematic meta-synthesis, BMC Geriatr 18 (1) (2018) 1–27.
[14] R. Khosla, M.T. Chu, S.M.S. Khaksar, K. Nguyen, T. Nishida, Engagement and experience of older people with socially assistive robots in home care, Assist. Technol. 00 (00) (2019) 1–15, doi:10.1080/10400435.2019.1588805.
[15] M.S. Sharif, M. Alsallal, L. Herghelegiu, An effective telehealth assistive system to support senior citizen at home or care-homes, Proc. Int Conf Comput Electron Commun Eng (iCCECE) 2018, 2019 113–117.
[16] D. Marikyan, S. Papagiannidis, E. Alamanos, A systematic review of the smart home literature: a user perspective, Technol. Forecast Soc. Change [Internet] 138 (June) (2019) 139–154, doi:10.1016/j.techfore.2018.08.015.
[17] O.S. Albahri, A.S. Albahri, K.I. Mohammed, A.A. Zaidan, B.B. Zaidan, M. Hashim, et al., Systematic review of real-time remote health monitoring system in triage and priority-based sensor technology: taxonomy, open challenges, motivation and recommendations, J. Med. Syst 42 (5) (2018).
[18] H. Singh, V. Pallagani, V. Khandelwal, U. Venkanna, IoT based smart home automation system using sensor node, Proc. 4th IEEE Int Conf Recent Adv Inf Technol RAIT 2018, 2018, pp. 1–5.
[19] B. Hibbeler, Pflegeheime Skandale statt Lösungen, Dtsch. Arztebl. [Internet] 41 (102) (2005) 1. https://www.aerzteblatt.de/archiv/48694/Pflegeheime-Skandale-statt-Loesungen. (Accessed 23 June 2021).
[20] Türk L. Pflege skandal in Augsburg: Wie koennen solche missstaende-kuenftig verhindert werden? [Internet]. Süddeutsche Zeitung. 2019 https://www.stadtzeitung.de/region/augsburg-stadt/politik/pflege-skandal-augsburg-koennen-solche-missstaende-kuenftig-verhindert-id181339.html (Accessed 22 February 2021).
[21] A. Nayyar, V. Puri, N.G. Nguyen, BioSenHealth 1.0: a novel Internet of Medical Things (IoMT)-based patient health monitoring system, Proc. International Conference on Innovative Computing and Communications, Springer, Singapore, 2019, pp. 155–164. http://link.springer.com/10.1007/978-981-13-2324-9.
[22] A. Bossen, H. Kim, A. Steinhoff, M. Strieker, K. Williams, Emerging roles for telemedicine and smart technologies in dementia care, Smart Homecare Technol. TeleHealth49. (2015).
[23] I. Rawtaer, R. Mahendran, E.H. Kua, H.P. Tan, H.X. Tan, T.S. Lee, et al., Early detection of mild cognitive impairment with in-home sensors to monitor behavior patterns in community-dwelling senior citizens in Singapore: cross-sectional feasibility study, J. Med. Internet Res 22 (5) (2020) 1–10.
[24] L. Patrono, P. Primiceri, P. Rametta, I. Sergi, P. Visconti, An innovative approach for monitoring elderly behavior by detecting home appliance's usage, 2017 In: Proc. 25th Int Conf Software, Telecommun Comput Networks, SoftCOM 2017, 2017.
[25] L.A. Guerrero, F. Vasquez, S.F. Ochoa, An indoor navigation system for the visually impaired, Sensors. (Switzerland) 12 (6) (2012) 8236–8258.
[26] A. Vitanza, G. D'Onofrio, F. Ricciardi, D. Sancarlo, A. Greco, F. Giuliani, Assistive robots for the elderly: innovative tools to gather health relevant data, in: S. Consoli, D.R. Recupero, M. Petković (Eds.), Data Science for Healthcare, Springer International Publishing, Cham, 2019, pp. 195–215. http://link.springer.com/10.1007/978-3-030-05249-2_7.
[27] J. Broekens, M. Heerink, H. Rosendal, Assistive social robots in elderly care: a review, Gerontechnology 8 (2) (2009), doi:10.4017/gt.2009.08.02.002.00. http://gerontechnology.info/index.php/journal/article/view/1011.
[28] D.G. Bruce, G.A. Paley, P. Nichols, D. Roberts, P.J. Underwood, F. Schaper, Physical disability contributes to caregiver stress in dementia caregivers, J. Gerontol. A Biol. Sci. Med. Sci 60 (3) (2005) 345–349.

[29] S. Sörensen, P. Duberstein, D. Gill, M. Pinquart, Dementia care: mental health effects, intervention strategies, and clinical implications, Lancet Neurol 5 (11) (2006) 961–973.

[30] C. Cooper, T.B.S. Balamurali, G. Livingston, A systematic review of the prevalence and covariates of anxiety in caregivers of people with dementia, Int. Psychogeriatr 19 (2) (2007) 175–195.

[31] C. Simpson, P. Carter, Dementia behavioural and psychiatric symptoms: effect on caregiver's sleep, J. Clin. Nurs 22 (21–22) (2013) 3042–3052, doi:10.1111/jocn.12127.

[32] B. Schoenmakers, F. Buntinx, J. Delepeleire, Factors determining the impact of caregiving on caregivers of elderly patients with dementia. A systematic literature review, Maturitas 66 (2) (2010) 191–200, doi:10.1016/j.maturitas.2010.02.009.

[33] K. Ornstein, J.E. Gaugler, The problem with "problem behaviors": a systematic review of the association between individual patient behavioral and psychological symptoms and caregiver depression and burden within the dementia patient–caregiver dyad, Int. Psychogeriatr 24 (10) (2012) 1536–1552.

[34] C.Y. Chiao, H.S. Wu, C.Y. Hsiao, Caregiver burden for informal caregivers of patients with dementia: a systematic review, Int. Nurs. Rev 62 (3) (2015) 340–350.

[35] M.M. Blom, S.H. Zarit, R.B.M. Groot Zwaaftink, P. Cuijpers, A.M. Pot, Effectiveness of an internet intervention for family caregivers of people with dementia: results of a randomized controlled trial, PLoS One 10 (2) (2015) 1–11, doi:10.1371/journal.pone.0116622.

[36] N.P.G. Boumans, E. Dorant, A cross-sectional study on experiences of young adult carers compared to young adult noncarers: parentification, coping and resilience, Scand. J. Caring. Sci 32 (4) (2018) 1409–1417.

CHAPTER

5

Telehealth for the geriatric population: uses, opportunities, and challenges

Dari Alhuwail[a,b]*, *Alaa Abd-Alrazaq*[c], *Eiman Al-Jafar*[d], *Mowafa Househ*[c]

[a]Department of Information Science, College of Life Sciences, Kuwait University, Kuwait, [b]Health Informatics Unit, Dasman Diabetes Institute, Kuwait, [c]Division of Information and Computing Technology, College of Science and Engineering, Hamad Bin Khalifa University, Qatar Foundation, Doha, Qatar, [d]Health Informatics and Information Management, Faculty of Allied Health Sciences, Kuwait University, Kuwait

LEARNING OBJECTIVES

After reading this chapter, you should be able to:

- Understand the different uses of telehealth including, telemonitoring and teleservices, in the geriatric population.
- Explore the benefits and potentials of using telehealth for providing care to the geriatric population.
- Discuss the major challenges associated with leveraging telehealth for the geriatric population.

5.1 Introduction

In today's hyperconnected world, the ubiquity of the Internet, and widespread of information and communication technologies (ICT), the practice of telehealth facilitates opportunities to improve access to health and care

*Department of Information Science, College of Life Sciences, Kuwait University, Kuwait.

Smart Home Technologies and Services for Geriatric Rehabilitation
DOI: https://doi.org/10.1016/B978-0-32-385173-2.00008-4

services and connects various health professionals no matter the distance. The World Health Organization (WHO) defines telehealth as the "delivery of healthcare services, where patients and providers are separated by distance." [1]. Telehealth uses ICT for the exchange of information for the diagnosis and treatment of diseases and injuries, research and evaluation, and for the continuing education of health professionals. While sometimes used interchangeably, telehealth and telemedicine are different. The American Academy of Family Physicians explains that "telehealth is different from telemedicine in that it refers to a broader scope of remote healthcare services than telemedicine. Telemedicine refers specifically to remote clinical services, while telehealth can refer to remote nonclinical services." [2]. Telehealth can contribute toward achieving universal health coverage through improving access to quality, cost-effectiveness, and health services to people no matter where they live; "It is particularly valuable for those in remote areas, vulnerable groups, and ageing populations." [1]. Telemonitoring, a form of telehealth, leverages ICT to monitor and transmit data related to an individual's health status and can enable healthcare providers to monitor patients in the comfort of their homes or assisted living facilities [3]. Telemonitoring can function as a surrogate to in-person encounters and hence can enable clinicians to diagnose and offer pre-and posttreatment care comparable to traditional face-to-face medical visits.

Worldwide, and at an increasingly unprecedented pace, the proportion of people aged 60 years and older is growing, especially in developing countries. The WHO estimates that in 2019 alone, people aged 60 and older were approximately 1 billion individuals and the number is expected to rise to 1.4 billion in 2030, reaching 2.1 billion over the next 30 years [4]. The off shoot of this is that the increase in the elderly population across the world has caused an additional burden on healthcare systems the world over. [5,6]. The rapidly aging population is associated with an increase in the prevalence of chronic diseases [5] and the associated functional decline, rehospitalizations, frequent emergency department visits, increase in the length of hospital stay, comorbidities, and loss of autonomy [7]. Older adults with chronic diseases, such as cardiovascular diseases, chronic respiratory diseases, or diabetes, often have complex healthcare needs and require intensive medical and social services to maintain their wellbeing and manage their health conditions. Accessibility to healthcare services is of great concern to geriatric patients especially those living in less fortunate conditions or rural areas, as difficulty in accessing services may put their health and wellbeing at risk. Therefore, introducing the use of ICT to communicate remotely with their healthcare providers is a valuable solution to easing the difficulties they would otherwise face in accessing care.

The challenges posed to healthcare authorities in the provision of care by the higher demands for "patient-centeredness and quality of care, amid restricted resources" [8] has placed the onus on healthcare authorities to find ways of providing alternatives to sustain continuity of care and meet elderly expectations [9]. One of the alternatives is the use of telehealth to facilitate access to health services to maintain physical and cognitive rehabilitation especially for elderly patients residing at their homes or institutional healthcare facilities such as nursing homes [10].

While every individual would age differently, one thing is certain: physical and mental capacity tends to decline with increasing age. As such, Healthcare systems around the globe have started to invest in and leverage various digital health solutions to improve access and the quality of care for the elderly; these investments are crucial to alleviate the growing demands of aging populations. Telehealth solutions can provide a new opportunity for diagnosing, treating, rehabilitating, monitoring, and educating the elderly from the comfort of their homes.

In this chapter, we discuss the various uses and examples of leveraging telehealth, including, telemonitoring and teleservices in the geriatric population. We will explore the benefits and potentials of using telehealth for providing care to the geriatric population and discuss the major challenges associated with leveraging telehealth in caring for the elderly.

5.2 Uses of telehealth

Facilities available through telehealth can empower elderly patients and help them to be more independent at home by providing them with several services, such as screening, diagnosis, consultations, treatment, education, rehabilitation, and monitoring [11]. The most common uses of telehealth for elderly patients are overviewed in Figure 5.1 and discussed in the following subsections.

5.2.1 Screening and diagnosis

Deterioration in the physical and mental health of geriatric patients' may begin years before the disorder is detected and diagnosed [12]. Thus, telehealth can play a crucial role in detecting such deterioration through prevention, early diagnosis, and/or providing treatment for geriatric disorders. Telehealth for elderly patients can be used to screen and diagnose mental disorders (e.g., dementia, anxiety, and depression), neurological disorders (e.g., Parkinson's disease and Alzheimer's disease), and cardiovascular disorders (e.g., hypertension and stroke). Several technologies can be used for telescreening and telediagnosis, namely: videoconferencing [13,14], telephone [15], sensors [16,17], conversational agents/chatbots [18,19], and virtual reality [20,21]. For example, videoconferencing technologies (e.g., Zoom and Skype) can be utilized for screening cognitive

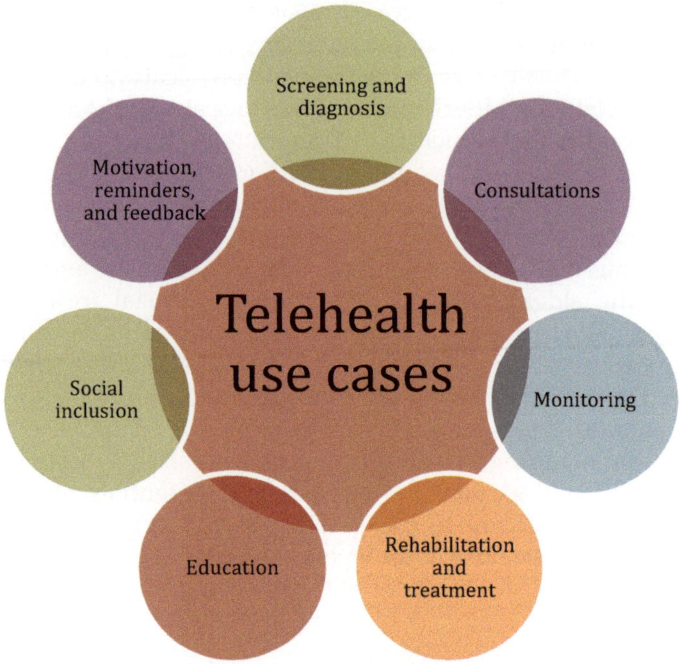

FIG. 5.1 Overview of Telehealth uses for geriatric population care explored in this chapter.

deterioration in survivors of stroke [22] and individuals with Parkinson's disease [23] and for the diagnosis of dementia in elderly individuals with memory issues [24]. Telehealth facilities can also be used to expedite the diagnosis of acute cardiovascular problems in geriatric patients; for example, through the immediate transmission of electrocardiogram data from a public emergency team to a cardiologist for prompt interpretation and diagnosis [25].

5.2.2 Consultations

It is well known that elderly individuals are more vulnerable to acute and chronic diseases, which require them to have more recurrent consultation visits to healthcare providers. Such visits are stressful, tiring, and expensive, especially for patients with physical and cognitive impairment [26]. Thus, telehealth is commonly used for providing consultations to the elderly. Teleconsultations can be synchronous (live interactive) or asynchronous (store-and-forward) [27,28]. Synchronous teleconsultations refer to consultations that occur between healthcare providers and healthcare provider through audio and video conferencing methods [27,28]. In asynchronous teleconsultations, geriatric patients send images, videos, and/or texts to healthcare providers via email or a web-based application. Healthcare providers, in turn, will review them and reply to the geriatric patient at their convenience [27,28]. Paul et al. provided palliative care teleconsultations for geriatric patients through mobile web-based video conferencing [29]. Furthermore, dementia clinics can provide a videoconferencing-based consultation service for patients with dementia and their caregivers [30].

5.2.3 Monitoring

Telehealth can be used for monitoring geriatric patients to detect functional decline or deterioration before their need for acute care in healthcare settings. Specifically, telehealth facilities can be utilized to monitor the vital signs of patients (e.g., heart rate, body temperature, oxygen saturation, and blood pressure) and their activities and behavior (e.g., falls, sleep patterns, caloric intake, syncope, and adherence to medical treatment) [5,31]. Furthermore, telehealth facilities can be used to remotely monitor and control the environment of the elderly for example, for the detection of smoke, gas leakage, overflowing sink or bath, unusual movement, as well as to control stove and oven, water and room temperature, lighting, intruder alarm, and door and window security [5,32]. Telemonitoring mainly depends on sensors (e.g., smoke and gas detector, flood detector, motion sensors, and fall detectors), medical devices (e.g., glucometer, spirometer, weight scale, and sphygmomanometer), and communication systems (e.g., Internet, wireless, Global System for Mobile) [5]. An example of a telemonitoring solution for geriatric patients is the SMARTA project [33]. The project aimed to monitor the health of seniors in their houses using a Bluetooth weight scale, multipurpose health devices for monitoring vital signs (blood sugar, heart rate, blood pressure, blood oxygen saturation, and ear temperature), a fall detection device, and environmental sensors for checking and controlling water tap, refrigerator, and dishwasher doors [33]. This telemonitoring solution notifies patients and clinicians in case of anomalies detected by the connected devices and sensors [33].

5.2.4 Rehabilitation and treatment

One of the most common uses of telehealth for geriatric patients is rehabilitation. Telehealth solutions are used mainly for rehabilitating older individuals with cardiovascular, neurological, orthopedic, and psychological problems [5]. Recent evidence suggests that *"interventions delivered using technology have shown better effects compared to traditional cognitive training and rehabilitation programs in improving cognitive function and quality of life."* [34]. In telerehabilitation sessions, the elderly perform exercises and activities based on video or direct instructions sent by the therapist online [5]. Usually, video game consoles are used (e.g., Nintendo Wii and

PlayStation Move) for telerehabilitation given that they are relatively less expensive, easy to use, and easily carried or moved [35]. TeleWii is an example of a telerehabilitation solution for postural instability in elderly individuals with Parkinson's disease [36]. TeleWii provides virtual reality–based balance training through the Nintendo Wii console, the Wii Fit gaming system, and a balance board [36]. A physiotherapist used a Skype video call to supervise the patient during the training session, which lasts 50 min [36].

5.2.5 Education

Elderly patients require education about their diseases, medications, risk factors, self-management, diet, symptom monitoring, problem-solving strategies, and so on. Telehealth facilities can be used to deliver education to geriatric patients at home [11,29]. Teleeducation can be delivered to geriatric patients in groups or individually. Schweickert et al. provided education about stroke to seniors through video conferencing [37]. I-TEAM is another telehealth facility that provides education about problem-solving strategies and behavioral activation for elderly patients with heart failure and chronic obstructive pulmonary disease [38].

5.2.6 Social inclusion

In addition to physical and mental wellbeing, social well-being is a main pillar of health as defined by the World Health Organization [39]. Social wellbeing in elderly people is more likely to decline due to increased isolation and lack of communication with others. Telehealth can enhance the social wellbeing of elderly people through providing social inclusion services, such as enabling/facilitating communication with friends and family members, traveling, shopping, socializing, learning, and interacting with the community [40]. An example of such telehealth solutions is MoveCare; which is a robot integrated with Smart objects, sensors, a virtual community, and an activity center [41]. In addition to monitoring the elderly and assisting them in activities of daily living (ADLs), MoveCare provides cognitive, physical, and social activities addressing their needs and habits to increase their social inclusion [41]. Indeed, one of such innovations is the robot "ROBIN" that has been developed to monitor seniors' health status and foster their social inclusion through communicating with their healthcare providers, friends, and family members [42].

5.2.7 Motivation, reminders, and feedback

It is crucial that geriatric patients comply and adhere to healthcare providers' instructions and prescribed treatment. Telehealth can provide motivation, reminders, and feedback for elderly patients to increase their compliance with treatments [41]. For instance, a robotic device was integrated into a telehealth system to increase medication adherence for older people [43]. The robotic device, which stores the prescribed medications, reminds the patient at predetermined dosing times via a voice reminder, a light signal, and written messages [43]. The patient, in turn, needs to process a dispenser button on the robotic device to get a sachet containing the medication [43]. If the patient does not dispense the dose, the telehealth system will notify the healthcare provider to contact the patient or visit his/her house to give the dose [43]. Another example is MyHealtheBladder; which is a mobile-based telehealth system for treating urinary incontinence in elderly women [44]. MyHealtheBladder provides 56 daily sessions about pelvic floor muscle exercises, bladder control, self-monitoring, risk factors, and a motivational quote after each session to motivate women [44]. Emails are sent daily to women to remind them to complete the sessions [44].

5.3 Telehealth benefits and opportunities

Telehealth brings numerous opportunities for the elderly to live and stay in their own homes as they age. Opportunities and benefits of leveraging telehealth for the care of the elderly are explored and presented below from the perspectives of geriatric patients, caregivers, and healthcare providers.

5.3.1 Geriatric patients

New technologies allow geriatric patients to maintain independent living and to safely reside in their homes [45]. In addition, the adoption of technology bridges the technological gap across generations by teaching elderly people how to use technology to assist them in performing ADLs, and in the strengthening of communication with friends and families [46]. Several studies have described the positive impact of assistive technology on elderly individuals in terms of empowering them, improving their quality of life and care, as well as their clinical outcomes. [45,47,48]. Using telehealth by geriatric patients assists in reducing the cost of face-to-face visits to their healthcare providers, hospital readmissions, emergency department visits, and travel/transportation expenses [49]. Telehealth facilitates convenient access to services for patients with limited accessibility, thus supporting self-management of chronic conditions. Telehealth can reduce the need for long trips to attend hospital follow-up visits, especially for those living in rural and remote areas. Additionally, telehealth can improve patient autonomy by helping them understand and control their wellbeing [50]. Some commentators have suggested that telehealth provides better follow-up, better doctor-patient relationship, better healthcare services, and encourages elderly patients to manage their chronic diseases [8]. Several studies related to the effectiveness of using telehealth technologies on elder patients showed a reduction in mortality rate, reduction in frequency of hospital readmissions, reduction in length of hospital stay as well as emergency department visits, and improved autonomy [51–53].

5.3.2 Caregivers

Caregivers are often family members or allied healthcare professionals and they provide physical and emotional assistance to patients outside formal healthcare settings. Caregivers help the elderly in performing ADLs and provide both emotional and social support. Looking after patients suffering from cognitive-related diseases, such as Alzheimer and Dementia, can aggravate caregivers' tasks [9]. However, using telehealth technologies, caregivers are able to easily access social support networks as well as knowledge sources to help understand the disease thus improve the patient-caregiver relationship, and decrease anxiety for both [54,9]. Caregivers can become more informed and empowered to support and care for their elderly in the comfort of their own homes.

5.3.3 Healthcare providers

The functionalities of telehealth can afford health and care providers' direct access to elderly individuals across geographical distances and in remote locations. By leveraging and using telemonitoring, healthcare providers can monitor the health data of patients in real time and analyze them. Additionally, providing the necessary healthcare services remotely via leveraging telehealth will minimize travel and transportation-related expenses for healthcare professionals and improve their productivity. Maintaining regular contacts with the healthcare professionals accelerates the diagnosis process, refills prescription medications, minimizes emergency department visits, reduces acute hospitalizations, and improves overall patient's quality of living [55].

Telehealth also affords health and care providers the potential to maintain rapport with their patients and allow them convenient access and direct communication with caregivers. The facilities afforded by telehealth have also opened new business opportunities in the healthcare industry by allowing healthcare professionals to expand the reach of their services to a wider population in various formats that is, as an individual, as a group of professionals, or a group of healthcare institutions.

5.4 The risks and challenges of using telehealth

The use of telehealth at home by geriatric patients presents challenges to some, especially those with physical and cognitive limitations [50,53,56]. These challenges can be due to different factors some of which are discussed in the following subsections.

5.4.1 Human factors

Technology acceptance—Elderly patients are vulnerable due to limitations in their physical and mental efficiency. For instance, those suffering from cognitive impairment such as Alzheimer's disease and dementia are usually dependent on caregivers. Therefore, acquiring new knowledge and skills may cause more stress, resistance, and anxiety for both the caregivers and the elderly patients [9]. In addition, limited digital literacy/technical knowledge and skills are generally considered as obstacles in the adoption of new technology by the elderly population.

Privacy, confidentiality, and security—Other concerns are related to health data privacy, confidentiality, and security. Privacy of patient information is a major concern because there is a high chance of putting patient's identifiable data at risk [57]. Further, there are doubts whether these systems and technologies can enhance the quality of care provided. Lack of social interaction and communication among older adults after using new technologies is of crucial concern to them. Adoption of technology means more interactions with devices and screens than human interaction [46].

Training and awareness—Healthcare authorities would need to conduct awareness programs about the positive impact of technology on patient care, clinical outcomes, independence, and improved quality of lifestyle of elderly patients [47]. Authorities would need to consider the provision of necessary digital knowledge, training, and education to all those involved with the implementation process including healthcare professionals, patients, and caregivers [47] as the provision of web-based access and online technical support would be necessary to increase knowledge, learn new things, and find information about chronic diseases. Also, the provision of technical support, counseling services, and patient and caregiver education will have a positive impact on technology acceptance [9,50]. Another success factor to be considered would be the provision of psychological support to patients, family members, and caregivers by allowing contact with health professionals [6,9,50,56,57]. Moreover, the active involvement of healthcare professionals would be required. Professionals would need to be equipped with skills, knowledge, and dedicated time to follow up with home-based older patients [48].

5.4.2 Technical factors

Ease of use—One of the main factors for technology acceptance by users is the ease of use [58,59]. Telemonitoring devices and teleservices should be user-friendly, validated, and approved by national and international regulations and standards [48]. Some commentators have also recommended the involvement of elderly patients, their families, and caregivers in the process of designing and developing technological applications to enable the customization of these applications to their needs [60,61]. In addition to developing the applications, developing instruction manuals including step-by-step procedures for using the system is of high importance. Therefore, including the perspective of users in developing the manuals will have a positive impact on their ability to use the system effectively [59].

Infrastructure and accessibility—Older adults should be able to access healthcare services including primary care and specialty care, whether residing at their homes, long-term care facilities (nursing homes), or in rural areas. Telehealth applications require using wireless sensor network (WSN) which allows elderly patients to practice ADLs at home or in specialized institutions, while their physiological parameters are monitored remotely [60]. The efficient use of WSN requires sufficient broadband connection and regular Internet connectivity. This might be difficult to accomplish for older adults living in remote areas, especially in developing countries that lack the necessary infrastructure to support new technologies [10,56,62,63].

Workflow integration—Another expectation is for telehealth technologies such as telemonitoring and teleservices to assist in patient care planning. Patient care plans should support care coordination, communication, and collaboration among different stakeholders, including patients, their families, healthcare providers, and those who have direct or indirect use of technologies. Integrating telehealth services into the traditional medical practice is not an easy task and the culture of the medical practice itself would need to evolve [6].

Cost and reimbursement—Implementing new technologies in the healthcare industry is associated with an initial high cost of technology equipment and training technical staff [62, 64, 65]. However, "upgrading and renewal costs become more cost-effective in the long term" especially after recognizing the new systems' benefits [66]. Geriatric patients are most concerned about the cost and reimbursement for using different telehealth technologies. Many emerging technologies are not covered by insurance parties, which makes it less likely for older adults and caregivers to use them [60]. Healthcare authorities would need to provide adequate funding to cover infrastructure expenses and recommend affordable plans to be considered by the health insurance parties to cover innovative technologies. Authorities would also need to establish a clear set of reimbursement policies to be discussed and approved by public and private parties and accepted to all stakeholders [10]. Collaboration among stakeholders from government, industry, and related not-for-profit organizations would be required to establish reimbursement policies, rules, and regulations to regulate the use of innovations in the provision of healthcare services.

5.4.3 Organizational factors

Legal and ethical considerations—Using telehealth in patient care would necessarily involve the integration of healthcare services provided by different providers. This means that healthcare providers would be required to set detailed guidelines for the development and implementation of a telehealth care pathway in the clinical workflow [48]. Commentators have described a lack of regulations for the provision of telehealth and there are recommendations available on the clinical, organizational, scientific, and ethical aspects [48] of regulations that would enable the smooth and lawful use of telehealth.

Clinical and organizational aspects recommendations included setting a clear definition of why telehealth such as telemonitoring programs, are used, evaluating patient's special needs, and determining the type of technology suitable for each case. Other regulation should cover data security, privacy, and compliance with legal and clinical guidelines such that patient data can only be accessed by authorized personnel. Examples of legal and ethical aspects recommendations are ensuring obtaining informed consent from patients on issues relating to their care. In addition to the above, given that the sustenance of healthcare would require, collaboration among stakeholders in government, industry, and academia [66], there would need to be a clear definition of the interface between these bodies including the licensing of physicians as well as any legal restrictions and the management of resources.

5.5 Conclusion

As we continue to witness and experience the rapid advances in technological solutions, telehealth brings major promises for enhancing geriatric care. Telehealth enables healthcare professionals to screen, diagnose, provide consultation, treat, educate, rehabilitate, and monitor elderly patients. Telehealth can also empower elderly patients to be more independent at home. As such, the facilities provided by telehealth are essential for the provision of comprehensive and high-quality health and care as people live longer with attendant complex health needs.

In this chapter, we overviewed various uses of telehealth for geriatric care and rehabilitation, explored the different benefits of leveraging telehealth, and discussed the major challenges associated with leveraging telehealth for the geriatric population. Telehealth as well as other advanced ICT solutions are here to stay and will continue to evolve. Leveraging them and integrating them into routine practice is a great opportunity to improve care quality and attain new levels of engagement with the elderly patients and their caregivers.

References

[1] World Health Organization, Telehealth - Analysis of third global survey on eHealth based on the reported data by countries, World Health Organization, 2016. http://www.who.int/gho/goe/telehealth/en/ (Accessed 16 December 2020).
[2] American Academy of Family Physicians. What's the difference between telemedicine and telehealth? https://www.aafp.org/news/media-center/kits/telemedicine-and-telehealth.html (Accessed 16 December 2020).
[3] A. Pandor, P. Thokala, T. Gomersall, H. Baalbaki, J.W. Stevens, J. Wang, R. Wong, A. Brennan, P. Fitzgerald, Definition of the decision problem. Home telemonitoring or structured telephone support programmes after recent discharge in patients with heart failure: systematic review and economic evaluation, NIHR J. Lib. (2013). https://www.ncbi.nlm.nih.gov/books/NBK260877/ (Accessed 13 November 2020).
[4] World Health Organization. Ageing. 2020. https://www.who.int/westernpacific/health-topics/ageing (Accessed 16 December 2020).
[5] M.M. Bujnowska-Fedak, U. Grata-Borkowska, Use of telemedicine-based care for the aging and elderly: promises and pitfalls, Smart Homecare Technol. TeleHealth 3 (2015) 91–105.
[6] R.C. Merrell, Geriatric telemedicine: background and evidence for telemedicine as a way to address the challenges of geriatrics, Healthcare Inform. Res 21 (4) (2015) 223–229.
[7] A.A. Zulfiqar, A. Hajjam, E. Andrès, Focus on the different projects of telemedicine centered on the elderly in France, Curr. Aging Sci. 11 (4) (2019) 202–215.
[8] J.K.B. Christensen, The emergence and unfolding of telemonitoring practices in different healthcare organizations, Int. J. Environ. Res. Public Health 15 (1) (2018).
[9] C.I. Martínez-Alcalá, P. Pliego-Pastrana, A. Rosales-Lagarde, J.S. Lopez-Noguerola, E.M. Molina-Trinidad, Information and communication technologies in the care of the elderly: systematic review of applications aimed at patients with dementia and caregivers, JMIR Rehabil. Assist. Technol 3 (1) (2016) e6.
[10] C. Hernandez, J. Mallow, G.L. Narsavage, Delivering telemedicine interventions in chronic respiratory disease, Breathe 10 (3) (2014) 198–212 Sep.
[11] W. Ludwig, K.-H. Wolf, C. Duwenkamp, N. Gusew, N. Hellrung, M. Marschollek, M. Wagner, R. Haux, Health-enabling technologies for the elderly—an overview of services based on a literature review, Comput. Methods Programs Biomed 106 (2) (2012) 70–78.
[12] M.C. Costanzo, C. Arcidiacono, A. Rodolico, M. Panebianco, E. Aguglia, M.S. Signorelli, Diagnostic and interventional implications of telemedicine in Alzheimer's disease and mild cognitive impairment: a literature review, Int. J. Geriatr. Psychiatry 35 (1) (2020) 12–28.
[13] A. Lindauer, A. Seelye, B. Lyons, H.H. Dodge, N. Mattek, K. Mincks, J. Kaye, D. Erten-Lyons, Dementia care comes home: patient and caregiver assessment via telemedicine, Gerontologist 57 (5) (2017) e85–e93.
[14] A. Carotenuto, R. Rea, E. Traini, G. Ricci, A.M. Fasanaro, F. Amenta, Cognitive assessment of patients With Alzheimer's disease by telemedicine: pilot study, JMIR Ment. Health 5 (2) (2018) e31.

[15] J.C. Mundt, L.M. Kinoshita, S. Hsu, J.A. Yesavage, J.H. Greist, Telephonic Remote Evaluation of Neuropsychological Deficits (TREND): longitudinal monitoring of elderly community-dwelling volunteers using touch-tone telephones, Alzheimer Assoc. Disord 21 (3) (2007) 218–224.

[16] T.L. Hayes, F. Abendroth, A. Adami, M. Pavel, T.A. Zitzelberger, J.A. Kaye, Unobtrusive assessment of activity patterns associated with mild cognitive impairment, Alzheimers Dementia 4 (6) (2008) 395–405.

[17] W. Amara, C. Montagnier, S. Cheggour, M. Boursier, C. Gully, C. Barnay, F. Georger, A. Deplagne, S. Fromentin, M. Mlotek, A. Lazarus, J. Taïeb, Early detection and treatment of atrial arrhythmias alleviates the arrhythmic burden in paced patients: the SETAM study, Pacing. Clin. Electrophysiol 40 (5) (2017) 527–536.

[18] P. Philip, J.A. Micoulaud-Franchi, P. Sagaspe, E. Sevin, J. Olive, S. Bioulac, A. Sauteraud, Virtual human as a new diagnostic tool, a proof of concept study in the field of major depressive disorders, Sci. Rep. 7 (2017) 42656.

[19] Ujiro T., Tanaka H., Adachi H., Kazui H., Ikeda M., Kudo T., Nakamura S. Detection of dementia from responses to atypical questions asked by embodied conversational agents. In: Proc. Interspeech 2018. p. 1691–1695.

[20] P. Allain, D.A. Foloppe, J. Besnard, T. Yamaguchi, F. Etcharry-Bouyx, D. Le Gall, P. Nolin, P. Richard, Detecting everyday action deficits in Alzheimer's disease using a nonimmersive virtual reality kitchen, J. Int. Neuropsychol. Soc. 20 (5) (2014) 468–477.

[21] S. Zygouris, D. Giakoumis, K. Votis, S. Doumpoulakis, K. Ntovas, S. Segkouli, C. Karagiannidis, D. Tzovaras, M. Tsolaki, Can a virtual reality cognitive training application fulfill a dual role? using the virtual supermarket cognitive training application as a screening tool for mild cognitive impairment, J. Alzheimers Dis. 44 (2015) 1333–1347.

[22] J.E. Chapman, D.A. Cadilhac, B. Gardner, J. Ponsford, R. Bhalla, R.J. Stolwyk, Comparing face-to-face and videoconference completion of the Montreal Cognitive Assessment (MoCA) in community-based survivors of stroke, J. Telemed. Telecare (2019) 1357633X19890788.

[23] T. Stillerova, J. Liddle, L. Gustafsson, R. Lamont, P. Silburn, Could everyday technology improve access to assessments? A pilot study on the feasibility of screening cognition in people with Parkinson's disease using the Montreal cognitive assessment via internet videoconferencing, Aust. Occup. Ther. J 63 (6) (2016) 373–380.

[24] M. Martin-Khan, L. Flicker, R. Wootton, P.K. Loh, H. Edwards, P. Varghese, G.J. Byrne, K. Klein, L.C. Gray, The diagnostic accuracy of telegeriatrics for the diagnosis of dementia via video conferencing, J. Am. Med. Dir. Assoc 13 (5) (2012) 487.e19-24.

[25] N.D. Brunetti, L. De Gennaro, G. Amodio, G. Dellegrottaglie, P.L. Pellegrino, M. Di Biase, G. Antonelli, Telecardiology improves quality of diagnosis and reduces delay to treatment in elderly patients with acute myocardial infarction and atypical presentation, Eur. J. Cardiovasc. Prev. Rehabil 17 (6) (2010) 615–620.

[26] L. Esterle, A. Mathieu-Fritz, Teleconsultation in geriatrics: impact on professional practice, Int. J. Med. Inf 82 (8) (2013) 684–695.

[27] R.E. Hoyt, W.R. Hersh, Health Informatics: Practical Guide, Informatics Education, lulu.com (2018).

[28] A.A. Zulfiqar, A. Hajjam, S. Talha, M. Hajjam, J. Hajjam, S. Ervé, E. Andrès, Telemedicine and Geriatrics in France: Inventory of Experiments, Curr. Gerontol. Geriatr. Res. 2018 Sep 17 (2018) 9042180. doi:10.1155/2018/9042180.

[29] R.L. Paul, C. Salmon, A. Sinnarajah, R. Spice, Web-based videoconferencing for rural palliative care consultation with elderly patients at home, Support Care Cancer 27 (9) (2019) 3321–3330.

[30] S. Dang, C.A. Gomez-Orozco, M.H. van Zuilen, S. Levis, Providing dementia consultations to veterans using clinical video telehealth: results from a clinical demonstration project, Telemed. J. E Health 24 (3) (2018) 203–209.

[31] M.R. Tomita, L.S. Russ, R. Sridhar, B.J. Naughton, Smart home with healthcare technologies for community-dwelling older adults, in: MA AlQutayr (Ed.), Smart Home Systems, IntechOpen, 2010, pp. 139–158.
[32] K.J. Turner, M.R. McGee-Lennon, Advances in telecare over the past 10 years, Smart Homecare Technol. TeleHealth 2013 (1) (2013) 21–34.
[33] L. Pigini, G. Bovi, C. Panzarino, V. Gower, M. Ferratini, G. Andreoni, R. Sassi, M.W. Rivolta, M. Ferrarin, Pilot test of a new personal health system integrating Environmental and wearable sensors for telemonitoring and care of elderly people at home (SMARTA Project), Gerontology 63 (3) (2017) 281–286.
[34] S. Ge, Z. Zhu, B. Wu, E.S. McConnell, Technology-based cognitive training and rehabilitation interventions for individuals with mild cognitive impairment: a systematic review, BMC Geriatr 18 (1) (2018) 213 15.
[35] C. Godinho, J. Domingos, G. Cunha, A.T. Santos, R.M. Fernandes, D. Abreu, N. Gonçalves, H. Matthews, T. Isaacs, J. Duffen, A. Al-Jawad, F. Larsen, A. Serrano, P. Weber, A. Thoms, S. Sollinger, H. Graessner, W. Maetzler, J.J. Ferreira, A systematic review of the characteristics and validity of monitoring technologies to assess Parkinson's disease, J. Neuroeng. Rehabil 13 (2016) 24.
[36] M. Gandolfi, C. Geroin, E. Dimitrova, P. Boldrini, A. Waldner, S. Bonadiman, A. Picelli, S. Regazzo, E. Stirbu, D. Primon, C. Bosello, A.R. Gravina, L. Peron, M. Trevisan, A.C. Garcia, A. Menel, L. Bloccari, N. Valè, L. Saltuari, M. Tinazzi, N. Smania, Virtual reality telerehabilitation for postural instability in Parkinson's disease: a multicenter, single-blind, randomized, controlled trial, Biomed. Res. Int. 2017 (2017) 7962826.
[37] P.A. Schweickert, C.M. Rutledge, D.C. Cattell-Gordon, N.J. Solenski, M.E. Jensen, S. Branson, J.R. Gaughen, Telehealth stroke education for rural elderly Virginians, Telemed. J. E Health 17 (10) (2011) 784–788.
[38] Z.D. Gellis, B.L. Kenaley, T.T. Have, Integrated telehealth care for chronic illness and depression in geriatric home care patients: the integrated telehealth education and activation of mood (I-TEAM) study, J. Am. Geriatr. Soc 62 (5) (2014) 889–895.
[39] World Health Organization. Constitution of the world health organization. 2006. https://www.who.int/governance/eb/who_constitution_en.pdf (Accessed 23 June 2021).
[40] M. Manzoor, V. Vimarlund, Digital technologies for social inclusion of individuals with disabilities, Health. Technol. Berlin 8 (5) (2018) 377–390.
[41] F. Lunardini, N. Basilico, E. Ambrosini, J. Essenziale, R. Mainetti, A. Pedrocchi, K. Daniele, M. Marcucci, D. Mari, S. Ferrante, N. A. Borghese. Exergaming for balance training, transparent monitoring, and social inclusion of community-dwelling elderly. In: Proc. IEEE 3rd International Forum on Research and Technologies for Society and Industry (RTSI), 2017, doi: 10.1109/RTSI.2017.8065964. 2017. p. 1–5.
[42] G. Cortellessa, F. Fracasso, A. Sorrentino, A. Orlandini, G. Bernardi, L. Coraci, R. De Benedictis, A. Cesta, ROBIN, a telepresence robot to support older users monitoring and social inclusion: development and evaluation, Telemed. J. E Health 24 (2) (2018) 145–154.
[43] P. Rantanen, T. Parkkari, S. Leikola, M. Airaksinen, A. Lyles, An in-home advanced robotic system to manage elderly home-care patients' medications: a pilot safety and usability study, Clin. Ther. 39 (5) (2017) 1054–1061.
[44] P.S. Goode, A.D. Markland, K.V. Echt, L. Slay, S. Barnacastle, G. Hale, M.K. Wright, T.R. Lane, K.L. Burgio, A mobile telehealth program for behavioral treatment of urinary incontinence in women veterans: development and pilot evaluation of MyHealtheBladder, Neurourol. Urodyn 39 (1) (2020) 432–439.
[45] R.G. Bozomitu, L. Niţă, V. Cehan, A.l.e.x.a. ID, A.C. Ilie, A. Păsărică, C. Rotariu, A New Integrated System for Assistance in Communicating with and Telemonitoring Severely Disabled Patients, Sensors 19 (9) (2019) 2026.
[46] E. Vaportzis, M.G. Clausen, A.J. Gow, Older adults perceptions of technology and barriers to interacting with tablet computers: a focus group study, Front. Psychol. 8 (2017) 1687.

[47] J. Ross, F. Stevenson, R. Lau, E. Murray, Factors that influence the implementation of e-health: a systematic review of systematic reviews (an update), Implement. Sci. 11 (1) (2016) 146.
[48] A.V. Silven, A.H.J. Petrus, M. Villalobos-Quesada, E. Dirikgil, C.R. Oerlemans, C.P. Landstra, H. Boosman, H.J.A. van Os, M.H. Blanker, R.W. Treskes, T.N. Bonten, N.H. Chavannes, D.E. Atsma, Y.K.O. Teng, Telemonitoring for patients With COVID-19: recommendations for design and implementation, J. Med. Internet Res. 22 (9) (2020) e20953.
[49] O. K. Burmeister, D. Ritchie, A. Devitt, E. Chia, G. Dresser, R. Roberts, The impact of telehealth technology on user perception of wellbeing and social functioning, and the implications for service providers, Australas. J. Inf. Syst 23 (0) (2019). [Internet]. https://journal.acs.org.au/index.php/ajis/article/view/1501 (Accessed 16 December 2020).
[50] N. Thilly, J. Chanliau, L. Frimat, C. Combe, P. Merville, P. Chauveau, P. Bataille, R. Azar, D. Laplaud, C. Noël, M. Kessler, Cost-effectiveness of home telemonitoring in chronic kidney disease patients at different stages by a pragmatic randomized controlled trial (eNephro): rationale and study design, BMC Nephrol. 18 (1) (2017) 126.
[51] K. Woo, D. Dowding, Factors affecting the acceptance of telehealth services by heart failure patients: an integrative review, Telemed. J. E Health 24 (4) (2018) 292–300.
[52] E. Andrès, A.-A. Zulfiqar, S. Talha, M. Hajjam, J. Hajjam, S. Ervé, A. El Hassani Hajjam, Telemedicine in elderly patients with heart failure, Geriatr. Psychol. Neuropsychiatr. Vieil 16 (4) (2018) 341–348.
[53] R.C. Walker, A. Tong, K. Howard, S.C. Palmer, Patient expectations and experiences of remote monitoring for chronic diseases: systematic review and thematic synthesis of qualitative studies, Int. J. Med. Inf. 124 (2019) 78–85.
[54] N. Nijland, J. van Gemert-Pijnen, H. Boer, M.F. Steehouder, E.R. Seydel, Evaluation of internet-based technology for supporting self-care: problems encountered by patients and caregivers when using self-care applications, J. Med. Internet Res. 10 (2) (2008) e13.
[55] H.K.Y. Almathami, K.T. Win, E. Vlahu-Gjorgievska, Barriers and facilitators that influence telemedicine-based, real-time, online consultation at patients' homes: systematic literature review, J. Med. Internet Res 22 (2) (2020) e16407.
[56] B.A. Clough, M. Zarean, I. Ruane, N.J. Mateo, T.A. Aliyeva, L.M. Casey, Going global: do consumer preferences, attitudes, and barriers to using e-mental health services differ across countries?, J. Ment. Health Abingdon. Engl 28 (1) (2019) 17–25.
[57] H. Ding, R. Jayasena, S.H. Chen, A. Maiorana, A. Dowling, J. Layland, N. Good, M. Karunanithi, I. Edwards, The effects of telemonitoring on patient compliance with self-management recommendations and outcomes of the innovative telemonitoring enhanced care program for chronic heart failure: randomized controlled trial, J. Med. Internet Res. 22 (7) (2020) e17559.
[58] K. Williams, P. Pennathur, A. Bossen, A. Gloeckner, Adapting telemonitoring technology use for older adults: a pilot study, Res. Gerontol. Nurs 9 (1) (2016) 17–23.
[59] B. Kramer, Dementia caregivers in Germany and their acceptance of new technologies for care: the information gap, Public Policy Aging Rep. 24 (1) (2014) 32–34.
[60] A.L. Bossen, H. Kim, K.N. Williams, A.E. Steinhoff, M. Strieker, Emerging roles for telemedicine and smart technologies in dementia care, Smart Homecare Technol. Telehealth 3 (2015) 49–57.
[61] M.A. McCaskey, A. Schättin, A.L. Martin-Niedecken, E.D. de Bruin, Making more of IT: enabling intensive motor cognitive rehabilitation exercises in geriatrics using information technology solutions, BioMed. Res. Int. 2018 (2018) 4856146.
[62] S. Sayani, M. Muzammil, K. Saleh, A. Muqeet, F. Zaidi, T. Shaikh, Addressing cost and time barriers in chronic disease management through telemedicine: an exploratory research in select low- and middle-income countries, Ther. Adv. Chronic. Dis. 10 (2019) 2040622319891587.

[63] S. Bhaskar, S. Bradley, V.K. Chattu, A. Adisesh, A. Nurtazina, S. Kyrykbayeva, S. Sakhamuri, S. Moguilner, S. Pandya, S. Schroeder, M. Banach, D. Ray, Telemedicine as the new outpatient clinic gone digital: position paper from the pandemic health system REsilience PROGRAM (REPROGRAM) international consortium (Part 2), Front. Public Health 8 (2020) 410.
[64] M.-N. Kouskoukis, C. Botsaris, Cost-benefit analysis of telemedicine systems/units in Greek remote areas, PharmacoEconomics 1 (2) (2017) 117–121.
[65] M. Akiyama, B.-K. Yoo, A systematic review of the economic evaluation of telemedicine in Japan, J. Prev. Med. Public Health 49 (4) (2016) 183–196.
[66] S.C.-I. Chen, Technological health intervention in population aging to assist people to work smarter not harder: qualitative study, J. Med. Internet Res 20 (1) (2018) e3 4.

CHAPTER

6

Smart home applications for cognitive health of older adults

Enrique Dorronzoro-Zubiete[a], *Octavio Rivera-Romero*[a,b], *Guido Giunti*[c,d], *José Luis Sevillano*[a,b]

[a]Computer Engineering School, Universidad de Sevilla, Seville, Spain, [b]I3US: Research Institute of Computer Engineering, Universidad de Sevilla, Seville, Spain, [c]University of Oulu, Oulu, Finland, [d]TU Delft, Delft, The Netherlands

LEARNING OBJECTIVES

- To provide an overview of current smart home applications for cognitive health for older adults reported in the scientific literature.
- To define evidence-based recommendations for designing smart home applications for cognitive health of older adults.

6.1 Introduction

The world is aging and that is a good thing. It means that we have been successful in fighting disease and improving the overall quality of life. The average life expectancy has surpassed the age of 80, and by 2030, it is expected that people over 60 will outnumber children under 10 [1]. However, reaching old age is associated with some issues. As people live longer, they also accumulate more health conditions that affect their daily life. Presently chronic conditions are the leading cause of mortality, accounting for more than 70% of all deaths, and with numbers projected to keep growing [2].

The need for health support services will continue to increase as the aging population sees their physical, mental, and social capabilities decrease. In the early stages it is often family members who act as

Smart Home Technologies and Services for Geriatric Rehabilitation
DOI: https://doi.org/10.1016/B978-0-32-385173-2.00007-2

informal caregivers to try to meet the needs of an older loved one, but more often than not, their own resources are not enough. Professional services are provided in healthcare facilities and nursing homes but the constant battle from both old adults and their families to remain autonomous and stay in their own homes for as long as possible is ever present. However, the impact aging has on cognitive skills such as memory, attention, problem-solving, and processing speed severely affects the chances of us keeping our independence. Getting old may not always be fun.

Recent research suggests that technology-driven interventions, such as Smart watches, monitoring devices, or locator devices, can help home care delivery and support the informal caregivers [3]. It has been shown that technology can help maintain independence and improve quality of life. Some examples of how technology can support older adults in living independently are: cognitive problems detection [4], tracking systems for dementia patients [5,6], training cognitive functions such as short-term memory [7], or augmenting human memory [8]. The interdisciplinary field of designing technology and environments for independent living and social participation of older persons in good health, comfort, and safety is known as gerontechnology [9]. Among these technologies, Smart homes, that can be defined as "a residence equipped with computing and information technology, which anticipates and responds to the needs of the occupants, working to promote their comfort, convenience, security, and entertainment through the management of technology within the home and connections to the world beyond" [10], are particularly interesting. Smart home applications (SMAs) offer a solution to the complex needs of the elderly and their families, monitoring physiological and functional issues, as well as aiding in emergency detection and response.

In the following sections we will provide an overview of the current state of the art in relevant topics and summarize the main findings into key takeaway points in the shape of recommendations.

6.2 Relevant issues in SMAs for cognitive health of older adults

6.2.1 Usability, accessibility, and acceptability

Aging is associated with changes that may imply several physical, sensory, and/or cognitive impairments [11]. Sensory and cognitive impairments might affect individuals' ability to perceive information, sustain and direct attention, memorize information, communicate, orientate oneself, execute activities, think and reason in an abstract manner, or understand and manage numbers and time [12]. Those changes impact negatively on their autonomy in the daily living activities. SMAs can assist elderly to perform their daily activities, monitor changes in their behaviors and condition, and provide digital training to prevent cognitive decline. However, to be effective, those applications must be designed considering their special needs and capabilities. Designers and developers must put a special attention in issues such as accessibility and usability.

Usability is defined in the ISO 9241 as "the extent to which a product can be used by specified users to achieve specified goals with effectiveness, efficiency, and satisfaction in a specified context of use" [13]. Evaluation of the usability of a technological solution comprises several aspects as it is defined in Nielsen's heuristic: learnability, efficiency, memorability, errors, and satisfaction [14]. Accessibility is defined in the ISO 9421 as "extent to which products, systems, services, environments, and facilities can be used by people from a population with the widest range of user needs, characteristics, and capabilities to achieve identified goals in identified contexts of use" [15]. Regarding cognitive accessibility, several standards have been defined by international organizations to guide the design process of cognitive accessible products [16–19].

Recommendation 6.1

The design process of SMAs for cognitive health of older adults must follow the current design guides for cognitive accessible products.

Good practice in the development of digital applications identifies usability as a key component [20]. Also, usability is included as a relevant criterion for the assessment of digital health applications in several standards such as the National Health Service Digital Assessment Questionnaire [21], the guidance from the Medicines and Healthcare products Regulatory Agency [22], or the Mobile App Rating Scale [23]. Undetected usability or accessibility problems affect technology acceptance reducing product adoption and user adherence and engagement with technology. Ensuring high usability may even result in increased accessibility. There are several usability testing methods ranging from qualitative (interviews, focus groups, heuristic evaluation, etc.) to quantitative techniques (questionnaires, task completion, etc.) [24]. It is common to use a combination of these methods in the usability evaluation of digital health applications. Most of these methods require the participation of target users in the evaluation. Involving people with cognitive impairments in the usability studies requires the adaptation of the specific techniques to their abilities and conditions. Examples of usability evaluation studies of digital health applications involving older adults with cognitive impairments have been found in the scientific literature [25].

Recommendation 6.2

SMAs for cognitive health must be tested following robust usability methods adapted to target users' abilities.

Interacting with technology might be a great barrier for older adults, especially for those with cognitive impairments due to their reduced abilities. In such circumstances, the device-free approach, that is focused on freeing users to intervene as little as possible, is becoming very popular in SMAs [26]. Following this approach, despite requiring users to carry any devices, those devices are located in the environment and capture the required information.

The methodology followed to design the technological solution has been reported as another relevant factor affecting technology adoption and user engagement. Due to the wide range of impairments that older adults can suffer, it is important to engage them and/or their caregivers in the development process of SMAs for cognitive health. Involving them may make easy to identify all potential barriers that would prevent target users from being able to use the application.

Several participatory approaches, such as user-centered design (UCD), have shown reaching higher user acceptance and satisfaction and lower user errors [27]. UCD proposes placing the needs and characteristics of end users in the center of the technological solution design and development, involving target users from the early stages of the process [27]. Following UCD ensures that digital health solutions are more likely to meet end users' needs and expectations. In addition, UCD defines an iterative design process that comprises four stages: Understanding the context of use, specification of requirements, solution design, and evaluation (find critical feedback on the product developed). Usability and user experience are commonly tested in the evaluation stage. As the process defined in UCD is iterative, the evaluation is performed from early stage of the development process, which allows to detect usability and accessibility problems early, saving time and money and decreasing design changes late in the process [28]. UCD has been used in the development process of SMAs for elderly [29]. Additional contribution of the design reported in the scientific literature is an increased level of accessibility to technology and a higher level of autonomy that users can achieve.

Recommendation 6.3

A participatory approach should be followed in the design and development process of SMAs for cognitive health involving stakeholders in the process. Both accessibility and usability must be considered and tested from the early stages in the development process.

Besides usability and accessibility, there are other factors, such as people's motivation to use SMAs and their perceived usefulness, that affect the acceptance and adoption of these technologies [30]. Older adults are more prone to show an initial rejection attitude toward the introduction of new technologies, and therefore, it is critical to examine those factors to understand what the utmost relevant factors are to be considered in new SMAs.

Studies on usability and acceptance of new digital health solutions for older adults conducted in laboratory or real settings are common in the scientific literature. Liu et al. reviewed studies on Smart homes and home health-monitoring technologies for older adults with complex needs published between 2010 to October 2014 [31]. This review is not focused specifically on applications for cognitive health, only 6 of the 48 included studies were focused on cognitive decline and mental health. The usability and technology acceptance were assessed in 32 of the reviewed studies, including all of those focused on cognitive decline and mental health, showing the importance of these issues. Authors concluded that acceptability and usability of the proposed systems were high among older adults based on the reported outcomes. However, they highlighted that none of these studies was based on theories that helped to explain intention to use and usage behaviors of participants. Usability evaluation is also a common test of SMAs in recent studies [32].

To fill the reported gap regarding the lack of theoretical basis of acceptance evaluation, several well-known and widely spread acceptance models such as the Technology Acceptance Model (TAM) [30], the Unified Theory of Acceptance and Use of Technology (UTAUT) [33], and their adapted versions may be considered [34]. Those models have been used as a theoretical basis in the technology acceptance assessment of digital health solutions in the ambient assistive living (AAL) domain [35]. TAM is a behavioral model of end-user acceptance of new technologies based on the Theory of Reasoned Action which states that the use of a system or service is based on the user's attitude toward it. In this sense, TAM proposes that perceived usefulness and perceived ease of use of a technology predict the intention to use technology, and hence its actual use [30]. Several studies have reported the influence of users' personal characteristics such as age, gender, cognitive abilities, or personality traits in the technology acceptance [31]. Subsequent iterations of TAM have included some of them incorporating additional factors such as social norms, technology experience, habit, age, gender, etc. [34]. Particularly, the Senior TAM (STAM) was proposed by Renaud and van Biljon [36] that included gerontechnology self-efficacy and anxiety, facilitating health conditions, cognitive abilities, social relationships, attitude to life and satisfaction, and physical functioning as factors that influenced perceived usefulness, usage behavior, and perceived ease of use.

Despite their wide use in research, those models are generic and relevant aspects in SMAs such as contexts of use, usage situations, or specific target user group are not considered. Hence, those models must be extended and specifically tailored to the specific SMAs and its functions. Biermann et al. conducted a study using an acceptance questionnaire adapted to AAL and the proposed technology [35]. Heerik et al. addressed the limitation of TAM that has not been developed for systems that can be perceived as a social entity, such as a robot, and proposed an acceptance model for assistive robots [37].

Recommendation 6.4

Acceptability studies of SMAs for cognitive health of older adults must be based on theories specifically designed for those target users and technologies.

Several studies have analyzed factors influencing technology acceptance and adoption among older adults. Liu et al. found seven factors impacting the perceived value of Smart home and home health-monitoring technologies reported by older adults [31]:

1. Participants stated that they were reluctant to accept the Smart homes and home health-monitoring technologies, if these technologies did not allow them to remain in their own homes and to age in place (user's preferences, Recommendation 6.3).
2. Technology must improve their quality of life to be widely accepted (perceived benefits, Recommendation 6.3).
3. Data privacy is identified as a critical issue in technology acceptance of SMAs (see 6.2.2.3 Privacy and security).
4. Inappropriate designs such as buttons too small on the touch screen, incorrect feedback messages, or level of false alerts causing distress to users (usability issues, Recommendation 6.2).
5. It is common that technologies under test are in their initial development stages, and thus, several aspects relevant for older adults are not still considered. (Recommendation 6.5).

6. The users' success with technology under study was associated with users' personal characteristics, such as age, gender, cognitive abilities, and personality traits (Recommendation 6.4).
7. Older adults consider some technologies as obtrusive systems (user's preferences, Recommendation 6.3).

Recommendation 6.5

The maturity of SMAs must be clearly informed to participants in evaluation studies, especially in technology acceptance evaluation. Also, the level of technology readiness to be used in target settings by target users should be indicated in scientific publications reporting evaluation outcomes.

Peek et al. studied changes and stability in the use of technologies by independent-living seniors [38]. They found a core of six interrelated factors closely linked to the frequency of technology use:

1. *Emotional attachment.* Perceived usefulness, engagement and satisfaction with the technology directly affects user's emotional attachment (Recommendation 6.4).
2. *Need compatibility.* Whether user needs are met using the technology. As we mentioned before, selecting a good design methodology such as UCD help to identify users' needs and creating products that meet them (Recommendation 6.3).
3. *Cues to use.* Users experiment certain cues that lead him/her to using the technology. In general, participants' cues to use could entail specific situations, routines, and places (Recommendation 6.6).
4. *Proficiency to use.* User's self-efficacy to use the technology. Learnability (ease of learning how to use it) positively impacts user's proficiency. Internal reward such as feel proud of being able to use the technology or reach a goal using it may also impact on proficiency. Sensory impairments could make difficult to use the application reducing user's self-efficacy. Hence, the importance of considering usability and accessibility as crucial issues in the design and development process (Recommendation 6.3).
5. *Input of resources.* Availability of resources such as money to buy the system or time/effort to learn how to use it. Perceived benefits of the use of the technology could positively impact these investments. Developing a usable (easy to learn) solution reduces time and effort (Recommendation 6.3)
6. *Support.* Finding help from others when user needs (Recommendation 6.6).

Recommendation 6.6

SMAs designs should assist older adults in the integration of the use of the application in their daily life. Accessible and tailored materials supporting older adults in the use of the application should be provided. Adapted cues should be showed on the user interface. Advanced features such as context-aware reminders/triggers informing on how the use of the application could benefit to users might be considered.

As it is mentioned before, the user acceptance of SMAs is influenced by user's needs and preferences and those factors could vary over time. Additionally, changes in physical and/or cognitive conditions could reduce the user's ability to interact with the SMA. In such circumstances, monitoring changes in user's condition allows automatically to adapt and tailor the SMA functionalities to the new context maintaining a high acceptance level.

Recommendation 6.7

User's conditions, needs, and preferences could be monitored, and the application must be automatically adapted when changes are detected.

6.2.2 Functionalities

Abdelrahman et al. analyzed the opinions toward information technologies, especially those for brain health, in healthy older adults living in an independent elderly living community [39]. They identified seven relevant themes reported by participants: physical activity, cognitive health, social engagement, organizing information, desire to learn new technology, advancing technology, and privacy/security.

6.2.2.1 Physical activity and cognitive health

There is growing evidence demonstrating the potential beneficial impact of lifestyle changes and cognitive training for overall health, and particularly for cognitive health. Several studies have reported the positive effects of physical activity and exercise-related brain stimulation to maintain memory and learning. Due to this demonstrated positive relationship between physical activity and cognitive health, including personalized coaching features in SMAs to support and motivate older adults to be physically active is interesting. These features should be designed considering behavior change theories and implementing behavior change techniques for physical activity promotion such as those defined in the CALO-RE taxonomy [40]. Additionally, personalization of these features may impact user adoption, adherence, and engagement. Therefore, designs of SMAs should consider personalization models defined for physical activity features such as that defined by Op den Akker et al. [41].

> **Recommendation 6.8**
>
> Designers of SMAs should consider including personalized coaching features to support and motivate older adults to be physically active.

Regarding cognitive health, there are three key applications for Smart home to increase older adults' autonomy:

- Monitoring of cognitive conditions and detection of potential cognitive decline. Behavior and health status recognition and subsequent transmission of collected data for remote monitoring.
- Digital cognitive training. Several studies have reported slowing down of cognitive decline, maintenance, and even, improvements of cognitive functions using digital training.
- Assistive technology that supports older adults in their daily activities. Common assistive technology functionalities associated to cognitive health are: Information collection, organization, and presentation; communication; location, navigation, and orientation; support in activities execution; and time management.

6.2.2.2 Social engagement

Social inclusion is a crucial factor in aging, especially when individuals suffer from cognitive impairments. Social isolation is seen as a public health issue for older adults that can affect negatively their physical, cognitive, and mental health. Technological solutions enabling maintenance of social relationships or improving social connections are more likely to be successfully adopted by older adults. In this sense, current studies reported that older adults use technology to socialize with their family members [39]. Also, these communication technologies enable an adapted alternative facilitating older adults and healthcare professional relationships. Not only communication, but also Smart home technologies enable remote monitoring that allows to detect critical events requiring healthcare professional interventions. Additionally, promoting social engagements facilitating social participation of older adults in community events reduces their loneliness feelings impacting positively their mental wellbeing. However, older adults are often less familiar with technologies and more prone to show an initial rejection toward its use. Some studies have reported mixed older adults' opinions regarding social features that highlight the need of individual customization, especially in people with complex conditions. Some facilitators for Smart home social technology adoption reported in the scientific literature are: ease to use and learn, training on technology use, and social features including customization.

> **Recommendation 6.9**
>
> SMAs should include optional and customizable social features adapted to user's communication ability and preferences.

6.2.2.3 *Privacy and security*

SMAs collect user information to monitor their conditions or behaviors and/or automatically adapt the system to their preferences and/or conditions. Therefore, privacy, data integrity, safety, and security are all strong requirements of these systems given their ability to collect and process sensitive information and make decisions based on this information. Hence, these issues must be considered in the development process of SMAs ensuring products and services are compliant with current regulations. In this sense, designers and manufacturers of SMAs should follow the privacy by default approach. As it is mentioned previously, privacy and security have been reported as relevant factors in technology acceptance by older adults. In some studies, older adults expressed feeling anxious due to loss of privacy, especially when cameras are used, and confidentiality concerns based on the risk of unauthorized access of their information. Due to concerns about this privacy invasion, and how end users would react to Smart home monitoring, some studies state that there is great variability in what factors about their life people would want to track, and that what people wish to track will change over time. Their interest will be based upon their age, life circumstances, interactions with friends and family, health status, and general curiosity.

> **Recommendation 6.10**
>
> Privacy and security issues must be considered from early stages of the development process of SMAs following privacy by default approach. Designers of SMAs should consider including personalization about the parameters to track and share. Including a clear and understandable privacy policy compliant with current regulations is mandatory when user data are collected, treated, or shared.

6.3 SMAs for cognitive health: study cases

6.3.1 Smart home architecture

A SMA generally consists of three layers: the *acquisition layer* that monitors the individual's context using a set of devices, sensors, and actuators (sensor platform); the *service layer* that processes, and analyses data collected to recognize the context of inhabitant and environment; the *application layer* that activates and deactivates services and helps make "visible" the Smart spaces to users [42]. Data collected by the acquisition layer are shared among devices, sensors, and actuator elements of the sensor platform and sent to the service layer using wired and/or wireless communication protocols.

The acquisition layer benefits from recent advances in embedded computing that have enabled the development of a huge variety of sensor and actuator devices that can be used in increasingly complex applications. These devices could be classified as: physiological sensors (heart rate, blood pressure, oxygen saturation, etc.), activity trackers, environmental sensors (thermostat, presence control, etc.), Smart objects (Smart fridge, air quality control devices, etc.), and advanced user interfaces devices (Smart glasses, social robots, etc.). Earliest Smart homes were composed of relatively simple nodes collecting information and transmitting it to centralized systems (perhaps in the cloud) for processing. The current trend is toward an Internet of Things model of powerful interconnected nodes (through wireless connections such as WiFi, 5G, or Bluetooth Low Energy) running sophisticated local processing (including advanced artificial intelligence) and sending this processed information (event data, alarms, recommendations, etc.) to central nodes, or even directly to the user.

The service layer includes advanced techniques to automatically recognize individual's cognitive condition, behaviors, and daily life activities performed. Artificial intelligence–based techniques to identify environmental elements that older adults can interact with are also included in this layer. SMAs use detected changes in user's condition to automatically adapt themselves to the new condition being responsive to users' needs and routines by predicting them instead of having to entirely rely on programmed routines. Additionally, healthcare professionals must be informed about these changes in conditions for early detection of potential mild cognitive impairments and events requiring intervention.

There are three key applications of Smart home for cognitive health that increase older adults' autonomy: Smart home cognitive health monitoring, digital cognitive training, and assistive Smart home technology. In this section, we present study cases representing some of SMAs for cognitive health published in the scientific literature.

6.3.2 Smart home cognitive health monitoring

Lussier et al. published in 2019 a systematic review of Smart home sensors technologies for early detection of mild cognitive impairments through the monitoring of everyday life activities [43]. They found 17 studies: 13 were conducted in real-life settings and 4 in a living laboratory. Studies conducted in real-life settings analyzed activities including mobility (walking frequency, walking speed, level of general activities, movements during nighttime), leisure time (computer usage), and self-care (medication uptake) while those conducted in lab measured time of completion, quality of activity completion, number of errors, amount of assistance needed, and task-irrelevant behaviors. Other systematic review, performed by Piau et al., analyzed the evidence for real-life home-based use of technologies for the early detection and follow-up of mild cognitive impairments or dementia [44]. Sensors used in the included studies were grouped into four groups based on technology (Table 6.1).

TABLE 6.1 Groups of sensors based on technology used to collect data.

Group	Sensor
Data from dedicated embedded or passive sensors	Infrared motion sensors
	Magnetic contact door sensors
	Radiofrequency identification
	Temperature sensors
	Driving sensor (passive sensing device plugged into participants' vehicle data port)
Data from dedicated wearable sensors	Sleep monitoring sensor
	GPS
	Inertial sensors
Data from dedicated or purposive technological solutions	Interactive voice response
	Personal digital assistant
	Touch screen system
	Online questionnaire/survey
	Augmented reality
	Nintendo Wii balance board
Data derived from use of nondedicated technological solutions	Electronic pill box
	Computer usage
	Mouse pointer movements

In a more recently published paper, Rawtaer et al. evaluated the feasibility and acceptability of utilizing in-home sensors to detect changes in behaviors of older adults as indicators of mild cognitive impairments [39]. Authors used a network of multimodal sensors delivered in participants' home that comprised passive infrared motion sensors, proximity beacon tags, a sensor-equipped medication box, a bed sensor (fiberoptic technology for sleep behavior monitoring), and a wearable (pedometer and heart rate).

6.3.3 SMAs for cognitive training

Traditional cognitive interventions are usually designed as group-based or face-to-face programs that require qualified therapists, appropriate facilities, and adequate locations for accessibility. The provision of these traditional cognitive interventions may be challenging due to the increase of aging population. Therefore, there is a need for innovative alternatives enabling cost-effective interventions. In-home digital cognitive training has been evaluated in the scientific literature reporting promising outcomes. Particularly, services robots can interact with humans offering appropriate services to provide home-based cognitive interventions. As an example, Lee et al. developed five programs for home-based cognitive intervention using a personal robot for people with mild cognitive impairments [45]. Authors used a robot named Bomy (Robocare, Seongnam, Republic of Korea) that provides five cognitive training programs focused on specific domains such as memory, language, visuospatial function, calculation, and frontal executive function.

6.3.4 Assistive Smart home technologies

In this study case, Microsoft HoloLens are used to enable users to interact with a Smart home in a project named HoloHome [46]. HoloHome creates virtual home appliances that are presented on the same position and scale alignment of the corresponding real-world objects. Each time the user moves his/her head and looks at a specific device through the HoloLens, additional information (images, animations, etc.) appears on that object to help using it. Examples may include a simplified control panel of the washing machine or hints to find ingredients in the refrigerator. The system is designed as an assistive tool for people with mild cognitive impairments suffering from memory and/or executive function deficits, improving their ability to perform daily activities in a more independent way.

6.4 Conclusions

We are only starting to realize what opportunities technologies such as Smart homes unlock for the care of old adults. Our modest success in extending our lifespan should act as encouragement for taking bolder steps to improve how well we live our life in the later stages. The world is aging, let us spend our golden years better with the help of gerontechnologies. We have presented an overview of current applications reported in the scientific literature. SMAs for cognitive health must take all listed recommendations into account, especially in the application layer design. The true challenge is to evolve from prototype implementations to fully useful, commercial solutions. Application development is probably the weakest part of current SMAs for cognitive health, and new approaches are needed that incorporate interdisciplinarity, personalization, participatory design, as well as standardization through technology-neutral abstractions of the lower layers.

Acknowledgment

Enrique Dorronzoro-Zubiete is supported by the "V Plan Propio de Investigación" of the Universidad de Sevilla. The present study is funded by the Fondo Europeo de Desarrollo Regional (FEDER) and the Andalusian Government from Spain (US-1263715) grant for the "Understanding Daily Multiple Sclerosis Related Fatigue: A Participatory Health Informatics Approach" (MSF-PHIA) project,

References

[1] Health at a Glance 2017 [Internet]. OECD; 2017. (Health at a Glance). https://www.oecd-ilibrary.org/social-issues-migration-health/health-at-a-glance-2017_health_glance-2017-en (Accessed 2021/02/25).

[2] WHO, Noncommunicable diseases country profiles, WHO, 2018. http://www.who.int/nmh/publications/ncd-profiles-2018/en/.

[3] K.M. Godwin, W.L. Mills, J.A. Anderson, M.E. Kunik, Technology-driven interventions for caregivers of persons with dementia: A systematic review, Am. J. Alzheimer Dis. Other Demen, Vol. 28, 2013 216–222. https://pubmed.ncbi.nlm.nih.gov/23528881/.

[4] Y. Zhou, Y. Lu, Z. Pei, Intelligent diagnosis of Alzheimer's disease based on internet of things monitoring system and deep learning classification method, Microprocess. Microsyst 83 (2021) 104007.

[5] C. Boletsis, S. McCallum, B.F. Landmark, The use of smartwatches for health monitoring in home-based dementia care. In: Lecture Notes in Computer Science (including subseries Lecture Notes in Artificial Intelligence and Lecture Notes in Bioinformatics) [Internet], Springer Verlag, NY, 2015, pp. 15–26. https://link.springer.com/chapter/10.1007/978-3-319-20913-5_2.

[6] P.P. Ray, D. Dash, D. De, A systematic review and implementation of IoT-based pervasive sensor-enabled tracking system for dementia patients, J. Med. Syst. 43 (9) (2019) 287. http://link.springer.com/10.1007/s10916-019-1417-z.

[7] L.P. Hung, C.L. Liu, J.Y. Shih, J.P. Wang, An innovative assisted living technology for short-term memory training at home, Proc. 2019 International Conference on Engineering, Science, and Industrial Applications, ICESI 2019, Institute of Electrical and Electronics Engineers Inc., 2019

[8] K. Gizaw, Neuroethics of augmenting human memory using wearable pervasive and ubiquitous technologies, in: K. Rannenberg (Ed.), IFIP Advances in Information and Communication Technology, Springer New York LLC, 2019, pp. 3–9. https://doi.org/10.1007/978-3-030-20671-0_1.

[9] Gerontechnology Journal. https://journal.gerontechnology.org/Aim.aspx.

[10] F.K. Aldrich, Smart Homes: Past, Present and Future. In: Inside the Smart Home, Springer-Verlag, NY, 2006, pp. 17–39. https://link.springer.com/chapter/10.1007/1-85233-854-7_2.

[11] K. Pottie, R. Rahal, A. Jaramillo, R. Birtwhistle, B.D. Thombs, H. Singh, et al., Recommendations on screening for cognitive impairment in older adults, Can. Med. Assoc. J. 188 (1) (2016) 37–46. http://www.cmaj.ca/lookup/doi/10.1503/cmaj.141165.

[12] WHO, World Report on Ageing and Health 2015, WHO, 2017. http://www.who.int/ageing/events/world-report-2015-launch/en/.

[13] ISO - ISO 9241-11:1998 -Ergonomic requirements for office work with visual display terminals (VDTs) — Part 11: Guidance on usability. https://www.iso.org/standard/16883.html.

[14] J. Nielsen, Usability Engineering, Morgan KaufmannPublishers Inc., 1993, p. 358. https://www.nngroup.com/books/usability-engineering/.

[15] ISO - ISO 9241-112:2017 -Ergonomics of human-system interaction — Part 112: Principles for the presentation of information. https://www.iso.org/standard/64840.html.

[16] Alr.Human Factors (HF); Functional needs of people with cognitive disabilities when using mobile ICT devices for an improved user experience in mobile ICT devices. 2016. https://progressivestandards.org/standard/human-factors-hf-functional-needs-of-people-with-cognitive-disabilities-when-using-mobile-ict-devices-for-an-improved-user-experience-in-mobile-ict-devices/.

[17] RESNA>AT Standards >cognitive accessibility (CA). https://www.resna.org/AT-Standards/Cognitive-Accessibility-CA.

[18] ISO- ISO 21802:2019 - Assistive products — Guidelines on cognitive accessibility — Daily time management. https://www.iso.org/standard/71712.html?browse=tc.

[19] ISO - ISO 21801-1:2020 - Cognitive accessibility — Part 1: General guidelines. https://www.iso.org/standard/71711.html?browse=tc.

[20] B.C. Zapata, J.L. Fernández-Alemán, A. Idri, A. Toval, Empirical studies on usability of mhealth apps: a systematic literature review, J. Med. Syst 39 (2) (2015) 1–19. https://pubmed.ncbi.nlm.nih.gov/25600193/.

[21] National Health Service. Digital Assessment Questionnaire V2.1. Nhs. 2018; https://developer.nhs.uk/wp-content/uploads/2018/09/Digital-Assessment-Questions-V2.1-Beta-PDF.pdf.

[22] MHRA, Human factors and usability engineering - guidance for medical devices including drug-device combination products, Med. Healthc. Prod. Regul. Agency (2017) 1–30. https://www.gov.uk/government/uploads/system/uploads/attachment_data/file/645862/HumanFactors_Medical-Devices_v1.0.pdf.

[23] S.R. Stoyanov, L. Hides, D.J. Kavanagh, O. Zelenko, D. Tjondronegoro, M. Mani, Mobile app rating scale: a new tool for assessing the quality of health mobile apps, JMIR mHealth. uHealth 3 (1) (2015) e3422. https://mhealth.jmir.org/2015/1/e27.

[24] J. Nielsen, Usability inspection methods, Proc. Conference on Human Factors in Computing Systems, New York, New York, USA, Association for Computing Machinery, 1994, pp. 413–414. http://portal.acm.org/citation.cfm?doid=259963.260531.

[25] M. Quintana, P. Anderberg, J.S. Berglund, J. Frögren, N. Cano, S. Cellek, et al., Feasibility-usability study of a tablet app adapted specifically for persons with cognitive impairment—smart4md (Support monitoring and reminder technology for mild dementia), Int. J. Environ. Res. Public Health 17 (18) (2020) 1–21. Sep 2. https://www.ncbi.nlm.nih.gov/pmc/articles/PMC7557766/.

[26] Z. Hussain, Q.Z. Sheng, W.E. Zhang, A review and categorization of techniques on device-free human activity recognition, J. Netw. Comput. Appl., Vol. 167, 2020 1–22. https://researchers.mq.edu.au/en/publications/a-review-and-categorization-of-techniques-on-device-free-human-ac.

[27] A.D.V. Dabbs, B.A. Myers, K.R. Mc Curry, J Dunbar-Jacob, R.P. Hawkins, A. Begey, et al., User-centered design and interactive health technologies for patients., Comput. Inform. Nurs. 27 (3) (2009) 175–183. https://pubmed.ncbi.nlm.nih.gov/19411947/.

[28] C.M. Johnson, T.R. Johnson, J. Zhang, A user-centered framework for redesigning health care interfaces, J. Biomed. Inform Vol. 38 (2005) 75–87. https://pubmed.ncbi.nlm.nih.gov/15694887/.

[29] E. Borelli, G. Paolini, F. Antoniazzi, M. Barbiroli, F. Benassi, F Chesani, et al., HABITAT: an IoT solution for independent elderly, Sensors. (Switzerland) 19 (5) (2019). https://www.mdpi.com/1424-8220/19/5/1258.

[30] F.D. Davis, Perceived usefulness, perceived ease of use, and user acceptance of information technology, MIS Quart. 13 (3) (1989) 319–339. https://www.jstor.org/stable/249008?seq=1.

[31] L. Liu, E. Stroulia, I. Nikolaidis, A. Miguel-Cruz, A. Rios Rincon, Smart homes and home health monitoring technologies for older adults: a systematic review, Int. J. Med. Inform. 91 (2016) 44–59. http://dx.doi.org/10.1016/j.ijmedinf.2016.04.007.

[32] K. Zsiga, A. Tóth, T. Pilissy, O. Péter, Z. Dénes, G. Fazekas, Evaluation of a companion robot based on field tests with single older adults in their homes, Assist. Technol 30 (5) (2018) 259–266. https://www.tandfonline.com/doi/full/10.1080/10400435.2017.1322158.

[33] V. Venkatesh, M.G. Morris, G.B. Davis, F.D. Davis, User acceptance of information technology: toward a unified view, MIS Quart. 27 (3) (2003) 425–478. https://www.jstor.org/stable/30036540.

[34] V. Venkatesh, H. Bala, Technology acceptance model 3 and a research agenda on interventions, Decis. Sci. 39 (2) (2008) 273–315. https://onlinelibrary.wiley.com/doi/full/10.1111/j.1540-5915.2008.00192.x.

[35] H. Biermann, J. Offermann-Van Heek, S. Himmel, M. Ziefle, Ambient assisted living as support for aging in place: quantitative users' acceptance study on ultrasonic whistles, JMIR Aging 1 (2) (2018). https://pubmed.ncbi.nlm.nih.gov/31518245/.

[36] K. Renaud, J. Van Biljon, Predicting technology acceptance and adoption by the elderly: A qualitative study, SAICSIT '08: Proceedings of the 2008 Annual Research Conference of the South African Institute of Computer Scientists and Information Technologists on IT Research in Developing Countries: Riding the Wave of Technology 338 (2008) 210–219. https://dl.acm.org/doi/10.1145/1456659.1456684.

[37] M. Heerink, B. Krose, V. Evers, B. Wielinga, Measuring acceptance of an assistive social robot: a suggested toolkit, Proc. RO-MAN 2009 —The 18th IEEE International Symposium on Robot and Human Interactive Communication, IEEE, 2009, pp. 528–533. http://ieeexplore.ieee.org/document/5326320/.

[38] S.T.M. Peek, K.G. Luijkx, H.J.M. Vrijhoef, M.E. Nieboer, S. Aarts, C.S. Van Der Voort, et al., Understanding changes and stability in the long-term use of technologies by seniors who are aging in place: a dynamical framework, BMC Geriatr. 19 (1) (2019). https://pubmed.ncbi.nlm.nih.gov/31462214/.

[39] Abdelrahman NG, Haque R, Polverento ME, Wendling A, Goetz CM, Arnetz BB. Brain health : attitudes towards technology adoption in older adults 2021; 9(1):23. https://www.ncbi.nlm.nih.gov/pmc/articles/PMC7823644/.

[40] S. Michie, S. Ashford, F.F. Sniehotta, S.U. Dombrowski, A. Bishop, D.P. French, A refined taxonomy of behaviour change techniques to help people change their physical activity and healthy eating behaviours: The CALO-RE taxonomy, Psychol. Health 26 (11) (2011) 1479–1498. https://pubmed.ncbi.nlm.nih.gov/21678185/.

[41] H. op den Akker, V.M. Jones, H.J. Hermens, Tailoring real-time physical activity coaching systems: a literature survey and model, User Model. User Adapt. Interact 24 (5) (2014) 351–392. https://link.springer.com/article/10.1007/s11257-014-9146-y.

[42] S. Helal, W. Mann, H. El-Zabadani, J. King, Y. Kaddoura, E. Jansen, The Gator tech smart house: A programmable pervasive space, Computer 38 (3) (2005) 50–60. https://www.cise.ufl.edu/~helal/projects/publications/helal_GTSH_IEEE_Computer_March_2005.pdf.

[43] M. Lussier, M. Lavoie, S. Giroux, C. Consel, M. Guay, J. Macoir, et al., Early detection of mild cognitive impairment with in-home monitoring sensor technologies using functional measures: a systematic review, IEEE J. Biomed. Health Inform 23 (2) (2019) 838–847.

[44] A. Piau, K. Wild, N. Mattek, J. Kaye, Current state of digital biomarker technologies for real-life, home-based monitoring of cognitive function for mild cognitive impairment to mild Alzheimer disease and implications for clinical care: systematic review, J. Med. Internet Res. Vol. 21 (2019) e12785. https://www.jmir.org/2019/8/e12785/.

[45] E.H. Lee, B.R. Kim, H. Kim, S-H. Kim, M.Y. Chun, H.K. Park, et al., Four-week, home-based, robot cognitive intervention for patients with mild cognitive impairment: a pilot randomized controlled trial, Dement Neurocognitive Disord. 19 (3) (2020) 96. https://pubmed.ncbi.nlm.nih.gov/32985149/.

[46] A. Mahroo, L. Greci, M. Sacco, HoloHome: An Augmented Reality Framework to Manage the Smart Home. In: Lecture Notes in Computer Science (including subseries Lecture Notes in Artificial Intelligence and Lecture Notes in Bioinformatics)', Springer Verlag, 2019, pp. 137–145. https://link.springer.com/chapter/10.1007/978-3-030-25999-0_12.

CHAPTER

7

From exergames to immersive virtual reality systems: serious games for supporting older adults

John E. Muñoz[a,b], *Maria F. Montoya*[b], *Jennifer Boger*[a,c]

[a]Department of Systems Design and Engineering, University of Waterloo, Waterloo, Canada, [b]HCI Group, Universidad Tecnologica de Pereira, Colombia, [c]Research Institute for Aging, Waterloo, Canada

LEARNING OBJECTIVES

After reading this chapter you will be able to:

- Understand the rationale behind the use of serious gaming that target older adults.
- Identify some of the unique challenges and opportunities of serious games for older adults.
- Become aware of tools and methodologies that can be used to create and evaluate player-centric games for older adults.

7.1 Introduction

Serious games (also called applied games) are interactive games that allow players to carry out activities that enable them to practice skills and achieve aspects beyond simply enjoying a leisure activity [117]. The rapid development of gaming technologies [1] (e.g., virtual reality, VR) is allowing researchers in the field of technology design for aging to engage in the exploration of a diversity of commercially available, highly motivating

[1]https://www.theesa.com/esa-research/2020-essential-facts-about-the-video-game-industry/

Smart Home Technologies and Services for Geriatric Rehabilitation
DOI: https://doi.org/10.1016/B978-0-32-385173-2.00011-4

serious games that can be used by older adults [80]. These applications may differ from those developed for younger populations. For example, serious games are often used as a complementary tool to existing best-practice methods to enhance users' engagement with activities that can be tedious or highly monotonous (e.g., physical activity, cognitive training, rehabilitation exercises) [69].

The term serious games for health has been used to refer to those activities that inherit game design elements (e.g., mechanics, story) to foster healthcare benefits [118]. Using serious games for healthcare purposes has been recognized as a valuable approach to engaging older adults in activities, particularly ones that can be monotonous, not very motivating, and/or difficult, such as repetitive physical exercises [66]. The adoption of games in healthcare settings is normally promoted by healthcare professionals who identify the potential of the technology as an opportunity to innovate in their intervention programs [53]. While the current literature supports the potential of using game-based training programs to stimulate both cognitive and physical abilities in older adults [106, 120, 121], research normally fails to demonstrate the effectiveness of such approaches because there is lack of more objective metrics to evaluate effectiveness as well as lack of more longitudinal, larger scale, and consistent experimental designs [86].

Interactive technologies that use games and digitally connected devices (e.g., mobile phones, tablets) have been promoted as a tool for assessment, rehabilitation, and early detection for both physical and cognitive conditions [5]. The goal of these technologies is usually to support nonpharmacological interventions to help maintain body and brain capacities through meaningful and enjoyable experiences that benefit physical and cognitive fitness [17]. Additionally, the ability for these types of technology to connect people from across the hall to across the world can be used to foster meaningful inclusivity that can mitigate issues related to social wellbeing and feelings of social connection [54].

Serious games that have been interfaced with motion controllers (e.g., accelerometers, cameras) allow for the involvement of parts of the body beyond the hands and fingers, which supports whole-body physical activity, while still having fun. This category is commonly known as exergames as it is a vibrant research topic in the field of serious games for health. Exercise has been shown to be beneficial for physical and mental health and plays an important role in fostering overall feelings of wellbeing. Engagement in frequent, effective, and timely exercise can help to mitigate age-related changes, increasing the possibility of having an independent and healthy old age [16]. While the benefits of participating in exercise are well documented, cognitive and/or physical changes that often accompany aging can make engagement in exercise more difficult for older adults and is a contributor to the increasingly higher rates of sedentary behavior with increasing age. With a growing global population of older adults, the exploration of innovative and emerging digitally connected technologies that can support aging is an important step toward creating effective, holistic solutions [76]. In addition to physical health, interactive and digitally connected technologies have tremendous potential to support recreation and social connectivity, which are important aspects to fostering feelings of wellness and quality of life [118, 54, 122].

The creation of virtual environments that use VR displays and interfaces is one of the most exciting trends in the field of serious gaming as VR provides a more immersive and believable sense of being physically present and a new paradigm of reality once compared with traditional nonimmersive technologies (e.g., 2D at screens) [99]. Commercially available VR equipment can be easily purchased and the evidence of its use in specific applications for assisting older adults is showing increasing effectiveness in well-matched applications, such as motor rehabilitation for upper limbs in stroke [52]. Despite growing evidence that customized, adaptive exergames (and other serious games) for older adults can be useful and motivating for exercise promotion and therapy, exercise practitioners still prefer off-the-shelf products (e.g., Wii, Kinect) [53, 54, 122], which have not been designed to take into consideration important aspects such as overexertion or cognitive impairments. The highest-rated barriers to the adoption of exergaming technologies were lack of funds, support staff, space, time, and appropriate clients [53]. More attention needs to be paid to the specific challenges and opportunities afforded by emerging technologies, including how to appropriately design and compare interventions intended to support end-users needs, preferences, and abilities.

This chapter emphasizes three main ideas with the aim of improving scientific activities and approaches related to designing and evaluating games for older adults:

1. Involve end-users and stakeholders early and throughout the design process to better capture real needs, motivators, and opportunities for using games.
2. Consider and complement the physical and cognitive capabilities of older adults when creating interventions, including the design of tools for evaluating user experience and effectiveness.
3. Custom-made, adaptive, and integrative gaming systems need to progress beyond exploratory studies to assess their impact in more generalized, real-world applications.

This chapter discusses facilitators and barriers to the design, development, and evaluation of serious games for older adults as well as ideas for engaging with and accelerating development of this new and promising area.

7.2 Related work

During the past 20 years, games for health have attracted the increasing attention of many industries and researchers due to their potential use in a wide scope of applications ranging from entertainment for young and exercising for adults, to clinical recovery in older adults. Older adults have been the central focus of several research teams that have seen the possibilities of using digital games to improve the wellbeing as they afford customizable access to activities in a way that aligns with a wide range of physical and cognitive abilities [46]. Different game modalities have been primarily studied with respect to the prevention of decline and rehabilitation of motor, cognitive, and cardiorespiratory functions in older adults [8]. Exergames were initially popularized by Nintendo and Microsoft when these companies created consoles that require whole body movements to interact with them (e.g., Nintendo Wii and XBOX 360) [118, 46]. Moreover, both custom-made and commercially available exergames in combination with traditional methods of physical activity have shown the potential of improving physical functioning in older adults. Exergames have been used to assess and monitor balance [8, 35, 47], mobility [81, 25], and general physical functional fitness of older adults [102, 41, 36]. Exergaming researchers are continuing to actively publish evidence to validate the use of exergames to support physical rehabilitation and training methods. While approaches differ, there is consensus among the research community that the motivation in older adults improves, in part, because games are presenting them with an attractive and challenging way of physical training [69]. However, there is no consensus regarding measurable healthcare benefits in aspects such as functional fitness, rehabilitation outcomes, and cognitive aspects among older adults [120]. One study concluded that with regard to cognitive function, both problem solving and reaction time were associated with arcade games and that overall playing digital games have the potential to be used as an intervention tool to foster older adult's wellbeing [128].

Other serious games applied in healthcare scenarios, such as puzzle or role-based games, have been shown to be effective in supporting the assessment of cognitive abilities across the lifespan, evaluating the underlying neural mechanisms, and providing cognitive enhancement [5]. Cognitive functions targeted by these types of applications are processing speed, attention, and immediate and delayed visual recognition memory [11, 9]. Some of these tools have also been used as preventive cognitive training for neurodegenerative conditions such as dementia caused by Alzheimer's disease and other dementias [88, 13].

Meta-reviews and meta-analysis have investigated the impact of using serious games to promote healthy lifestyles. These reviews have shown an overall positive affect in the use of serious games in multiple populations, for example: (1) exergames can be effective in and have positive impacts on healthy lifestyles and their determinants (e.g., attitudes, knowledge, skills) [123], (2) exergames are highly flexible and valuable tools for the rehabilitation and therapy of both motor and cognitive functions in adult populations with neurological disabilities [124], and (3) exergames were found useful to improve balance and mobility in older adults without neurological disorders, and to motivate patients to adhere to the balance exercises [125, 126].

While progress in the field of serious exergames is growing rapidly and shows promise, future research with longer studies and a greater number of participants need to be done to explore efficacy, better understand the impact of this approach, and to support more targeted development.

7.3 Design frameworks

As it is a relatively new and diverse area, designing a truly engaging and effective gamified solution targeting older adults is a creative process as much as it is following procedures. There are several approaches that are being used and refined to support the required considerations and systems involved in exergame design and development. This section discusses key frameworks that can be used in the creation of exergames for older adults. We start by examining three established approaches to design: (1) conventional design, (2) user-centered design (UCD), and (3) multidisciplinary design. These approaches can be overlapping, particularly in the case of user-centered and multidisciplinary design.

7.3.1 Conventional design

Conventional design methods are used to develop new software tools and games that often involve end-users only in the last stages of the design, usually to test prototypes [1]. Conventional design methods for designing games to foster physical activity and promote an enjoyable/fun rehabilitation in the aged population can fail to capture real needs and motivators, which in turn leads to problems in usability and adoption. Some of the disadvantages of conventional design methods are: (1) not including older adults early in their design process; (2) heavily influenced by new trends in gaming technology (e.g., VR, novel interfaces) rather than previous research in what has been used and adopted by professionals and older adults; (3) scope is tied to the length of the funding/research project and technology uptake is very limited, and (4) few (if any) iterations of the game are done with older adults.

The focus of quick-turnaround and focus on advancing technology capabilities tend to result in conventional design deprioritizing the importance of multidisciplinary collaboration and broad testing of the validity of their product. This amalgam of factors can lead to games that are not tailored to older adults or solutions that are difficult to be adopted in care homes or hospitals due to the impracticality of the technology used or the proposed interaction [28].

7.3.2 User-centered design

A *UCD* approach prioritizes ensuring the product (e.g., exergames) aligns with the needs, wants, and goals of targeted user(s). UCD involves end-users early in the process and consults with them often using a variety of methods such as focus groups, interviews, observations, and playtest sessions [14]. Indeed, most UCD approaches focus on having the target users identifying the problem, cocreating solutions, and defining what constitutes successful outcomes. UCD recognizes that there may be multiple end-user types, each of whom has different interests or roles. In the case of exergames for older adults, end-users could include older adults, exercise therapists, friends, and family members. Exploring the perspectives of the different populations that will interact with the exergame throughout its development helps to understand, capture, and design for users' reality rather than what the exergame creators imagine people might want [28]. This approach is also known as a player-centric approach where the design decistions are made by focusing on the player's needs, reactions and desires.

7.3.3 Multidisciplinary design

Creating effective exergames that complement multiple user types requires knowledge and engagement from multiple disciplines. *Multidisciplinary design* specifically focuses on the inclusion and interaction of multiple perspectives, including disciplines, levels of expertise, and sectors. The development team often consists of members from areas such as computer science, human factors/human-computer interaction, exercise therapy, gerontology, and (increasingly) representative end-users. Working as a multidisciplinary team requires creating a shared vision of the exergame and its goals, which in turn requires a consolidated commitment to creating shared vocabulary, excellent communication, and good working relationships [12]. The effort to support a multidisciplinary approach is rewarded with solutions that better reflect real needs in a way that provides legitimate value [56]. Therefore, multidisciplinary design focuses on gathering multiple perspectives, opinions, and experiences from a diverse group of experts, end-users, and other stakeholders to create a more informed and complete picture of the context and goals of the game. Multidisciplinary design usually uses player-centric design elements to enrich the knowledge of the target audience.

7.4 Evaluating serious games for older adults

The evaluation of serious games for older adults, and, in particular, exergames has multiple complexities associated with the: (1) heterogeneity of older adults, and (2) the lack of validated, aging-friendly evaluation tools in domains such as usability, game experience, and immersion. The objective evaluation of the benefits of digital games used by older adults has been carried out using several methods, most of them involving standardized questionnaires and clinical assessments.

In terms of physical and functional fitness, the benefits for older adults are associated with the improvement of the mobility [21, 102] and postural stability [8, 46, 69]. Improvements are measured through different physical tests such as the senior fitness test (SFT), the Time Up and Go test (TUG), Borg's scale and the Mini- Balance Evaluation Systems Test (Mini-BESTest). Few studies have investigated other methods for objective quantification of exergame performance [10, 9, 11, 36, 8, 107].

Cognitive benefits associated with the use of serious games are usually measured by their impact on (the improvement of) attention and memory. The most popular cognitive tests used by the researchers are the Mini-Mental State Examination (MMSE) and the Montreal Cognitive Assessment (MoCA), which are rapid instruments that assess orientation, attention, memory among other executive functions [109]. The MMSE and MoCA were both created for clinicians to perform a quick estimate of one's cognitive abilities. As such, these tests are not intended for measuring outcomes or impact of interventions and they lack the precision to understand how an intervention may be impacting the people being tested.

Quality of life is one's subjective perception of how good their life is and is a complex construct of aspects such as their physical health, psychological state, social status/relationships, and interactions with their environments [55]. Quality of life can be measured through validated questionnaires such as the Medical Outcomes Study Short Forms (SF-36 and SF-12) and the Quality of Well-Being Scale [18, 93], which have been extensively used to assess impact games for older adults.

Appendix 1 gives an (open source and shareable) overview of tools that have been used to evaluate multiple human factors when using serious games for older adults; a summarized version can be seen in Table 7.1. Table 7.1 presents 17 questionnaires that are often used in serious game design for older adults, which are arranged in five domains: (1) Usability, (2) VR, (3) Game experience, (4) Physical activity, and (5) Cognitive assessment. For each domain we describe the sample population, the technology used in the research, and the frequency of assessment for each questionnaire.

APPENDIX 1

Domain	Questionnaires/ Assestment	Descrption	References	Sample population	Assessment frequency	Technology	Availability		
Usability	System Usability Scale (SUS): Test domain: perceived usability	It consists of a 10 item questionnaire with five response options for respondents; from Strongly agree to Strongly disagree. It allows you to evaluate a wide variety of products and services, including hardware, software, mobile devices, websites and applications.	S. Nikitina, D. Didino, M. Baez, F. Casati, Feasibility of virtual tablet-based group exercise among older adults in Siberia: findings from two pilot trials, JMIR Mhealth UHealth 6 (2) (2018) e40.	60 OA (age range = 59–83) with non-to-mild frailty	post (after 8 week of protocol intervention, 3 sessions per week)	D: Tablet. I: Tablet touchpad	yes, online for free, not TUA	https://www.usability.gov/how-to-and-tools/resources/templates/system-usability-scale-sus.html	
			E. Pedroli, L. Greci, D. Colombo, S. Serino, P. Cipresso, S. Arlati, M. Mondellini, L. Boilini, V. Giussani, K. Goulene, et al., Characteristics, usability, and users experience of a system combining cognitive and physical therapy in a virtual environment: posi-tive bike, Sensors 18 (7) (2018) 2343.	5 OA (mean age = 70, SD = 11.70) without problems that prevent riding and without dementia	post (after one session of protocol intervention)	D: CAVE. I: cycle-ergometer			

			G. Corno, S. Bouchard, H. Forget, Usability assessment of the virtual multitasking test (V-MT) for elderly people, Annu. Rev. Cyberther. Telemed. 199 (2014) 168–172.	10 OA (age > 60) without any diagnosis of cognitive impairment.	post (after one session of protocol interven-tion)	D: HMD, CAVE-like. I: HMD controllers			
			T. Vanbellingen, S.J. Filius, T. Ny eler, E.E. van Wegen, Usability of videogame-based dexterity training in the early rehabilitation phase of stroke patients: a pilot study, Front. Neurol. 8 (2017) 654.	13 OA (mean age = 68.2, SD = 17.5) post-stroke patients	each session (after each session of interven-tion protocol of 9 sessions of 30 min, 3 times per week)	D: DC. I: Leap Motion Controller			
			A.G. Money, A. Atwal, E. Boyce, S. Gaber, S. Windeatt, K. Alexandrou, Falls sensei: a serious 3D exploration game to enable the detection of extrinsic home fall hazards for older adults, BMC Med. Inform. Decis. Mak. 19 (1) (2019) 85.	15 healthy OA (age range = 50–70)	post (after one session of protocol interven-tion)	D: DC, I: Mouse			

(continued)

APPENDIX 1 (Cont'd)

Domain	Questionnaires/ Assestment	Descrption	References	Sample population	Assessment frequency	Technology	Availability		
			Z. Saenz-de Urturi, B. Garc a Zapirain, A. Mendez Zorrilla, Elderly user experience to improve a kinect-based game playability, Behav. Inf. Technol. 34 (11) (2015) 1040–1051.	14 OA (mean age = 81.28, SD = 8.94) with mixed age-related disabilities	each session (3 sessions in 3 different weeks)	D: DC. I: MK			
			C., Boletsis, S., McCallum: Augmented reality cubes for cognitive gaming: preliminary usability and game experience testing, International journal of serious games, 3 (1) (2016) 3–18	5 OA (mean age: 67.6, SD: 5.77, range: 61–75) CPNR	post (after 2-month interve-tion protocol at an open and free rate)	D: Tablet, I: AR cubes and Tablet touchpad			
			M. Adcock, F. Sonder, A. Schattin, F. Gennaro, E.D. de Bruin, A usability study of a multicomponent video game-based training for older adults, Eur. Rev. Aging Phys. Activ. 17 (1) (2020) 3.	21 healthy OA (mean age = 71.4, SD = 5.8 years, Range: 65–91)	during-post (after 3 sessions and after a 7 weeks interven-tion protocol, 3 sessions per week)	D: Tv Screen. I: 4 IMUs and PC			

			T.E. Shubert, J. Basnett, A. Chokshi, M. Barrett, R. Komat-ireddy, Are virtual rehabilitation technologies feasible models to scale an evidence-based fall prevention program? A pilot study using the kinect camera, JMIR Rehabil. Assist. Technol. 2 (2) (2015) e10.	21 OA (mean age = 69.2, SD = 5.8) with mixed chronic diseases (no neurodegenerative)	post (after a a 90-minute session of interven-tion protocol)	D: PC. I: MK			
	Ad-hoc usability questionnaire	Questionnaires created by the authors based on previous Usability test, These question-naires have four main parts: PC experience, UX with HDM, UX with desktop and Comparing platforms	A. Plechata, V. Sahula, D. Fayette, I. Fajnerova, Age-related differences with immersive and non-immersive virtual reality in memory assessment, Front. Psychol. 10 (2019) 1330.	36 OA cognitively healthy (mean age = 69.47, SD = 7.39) vs. 25 healthy YA (mean age = 25.4, SD = 5.13)	during-post (after perform-ing the first task and after perform-ing the second task, in one session of 2 task interven-tion protocol)	D: HTC VIVE. I: DC	Yes, paper supple-mentary material, not TUA	https://www.frontiersin.org/articles/10.3389/fpsyg.2019.01330/full#supplementary-material	

(continued)

APPENDIX 1 (Cont'd)

Domain	Questionnaires/ Assestment	Descrption	References	Sample population	Assessment frequency	Technology	Availability		
		A usability questionnaire for the designed audio-visual content paradigm and look, tracking system, and acceptance of the developed system.	G. Epelde, E. Carrasco, S. Rajasekharan, J.M. Jimenez, K. Vivanco, I. Gomez-Fraga, X. Valencia, J. Florez, J. Abascal, Universal remote delivery of rehabilitation: validation with seniors' joint rehabilitation therapy, Cybern. Syst. 45 (2) (2014) 109–122.	19 OA (mean age = 69.31; SD = 7.38), with knee replacement	post (after 4 sessions of interve-tion protocol, pro-grammed for different days)	D: TV. I: inertial sensors and DC	No		
		A multiple-choice questionnaire constructed according to ISO DIS 9241-11 (21). Three questions regarding effectiveness (concentration on the task, alertness), satisfaction with the 3D-device, and efficiency (effort to learn and use) were answered.	H. Fordell, K. Bodin, G. Bucht, J. Malm, A virtual reality test battery for assessment and screening of spatial neglect, Acta Neurol. Scand. 123 (3) (2011) 167–174.	31 OA (mean = 74,1, SD = 11 years old), post-stroke patients	post (after one session of interven-tion protocol)	D: 19 CRT monitor and shutter glasses. I: DC, head-phones, robotic pen and keyboard .	No		

	User Experience Questionnaire (**UEQ**). Test domains: efficiency, perspicuity, dependability, originality, and stimulation.	The scales of the questionnaire cover a comprehensive impression of user experience. Is a survey of 26 consisting of 26 contrarian adjective pairs and participants rate each item on a 7-point Likert scale	L. Desteghe, K. Kluts, J. Vijgen, P. Koopman, D. Dilling-Boer, J. Schurmans, P. Dendale, H. Heidbuchel, The health buddies app as a novel tool to improve adherence and knowledge in atrial fibrillation patients: a pilot study, JMIR MHealth UHealth 5 (7) (2017) e98.	15 atrial fibrillation patients (mean age = 69.2, SD = 3.7).	post (after 3-month of constant use of the applica-tion)	D: tablet and mobile phone. I: tablet and mobile phone touchpad	yes, online for free, not TUA	https://www.ueq-online.org/	
			J. Gerlowska, U. Skrobas, K. Grabowska-Aleksand-rowicz, A. Korchut, S. Szklener, D. Szczesniak-Stanczyk, D. Tzovaras, K. Rejdak, Assessment of perceived attractive-ness, usability, and societal impact of a multimodal robotic assistant for aging patients with memory impairments, Front. Neurol. 9 (2018) 392.	10 healthy OA and 8 OA with mild cognitive impairments (MCI) (Range 60–81 years old)	post (after one session of interven-tion protocol)	D: Tablet. I: Robotic assistant prototype			

(continued)

APPENDIX 1 (Cont'd)

Domain	Questionnaires/ Assestment	Descrption	References	Sample population	Assessment frequency	Technology	Availability	
			S. Macis, D. Loi, A. Ulgheri, D. Pani, G. Solinas, S. La Manna, V. Cestone, D. Guerri, L. Ra o, Design and usability assessment of a multi-device SOA-based telecare framework for the elderly, IEEE J. Biomed. Health Inform. 24 (1) (2019) 268–279.	19 independely living OA (mean aged = 73, SD = 6 years, Range: 65–87) independely living	post (after 4 months of constant use of the applica- tion)	D: TV and Tablet. I: TV controller and Tablet touchpad		
Virtual reality	simulator Sickness questionnaire (SSQ). Test domains: Nausea, Oculomotor and Disorientation	Measurement of cybersickness' severity. This questionnaire contains 16 symptoms associated to cybersickness that are rated in a 0-3 scale.	G. Corno, S. Bouchard, H. Forget, Usability assessment of the virtual multitasking test (V-MT) for elderly people, Annu. Rev. Cyberther. Telemed. 199 (2014) 168–172.	10 OA (age > 60) without any diagnosis of cognitive impairment.	post (after one session of protocol interven- tion)	D: HMD, CAVE- like. I: HMD controllers	yes, online for free, not TUA	https://conservancy.umn.edu/bitstream/handle/11299/201892/SSQ%20Scoring.pdf?sequence=9&isAllowed=y

			B. Keshavarz, R. Ramkhalawansingh, B. Haycock, S. Shahab, J. Campos, Comparing simulator sickness in younger and older adults during simulated driving under different multisensory conditions, Transp. Res. F Traffic Psychol. Behav. 54 (2018) 47–62.	58 YA (aged 18–35) and 63 OA (age 65+), normal state of health	post (after every task in one session of interven-tion protocol)	D: digital speedom-eter displayed and Samsung Galaxy tablet. I: Logitech G27 steering wheel, gas and brake pedals, and Samsung Galaxy tablet touchpad			
			H. Huygelier, B. Schraepen, R. van Ee, V.V. Abeele, C.R. Gillebert, Acceptance of immersive head-mounted virtual reality in older adults, Sci. Rep. 9 (1) (2019) 1–12.	72 OA (mean age=74.8, SD= 10.4, Range: 60–92) CPNR	post (after one session of protocol interven-tion)	D: Oculus Rift HMD, I: Oculus Rift controllers and PC			

(continued)

APPENDIX 1 (Cont'd)

Domain	Questionnaires/ Assestment	Descrption	References	Sample population	Assessment frequency	Technology	Availability		
			J.S. McGee, C. van der Zaag, J.G. Buckwalter, M. Thiebaux, A. Van Rooyen, U. Neumann, D. Sisemore, A.A. Rizzo, Issues for the assessment of visuospatial skills in older adults using virtual environment technology, CyberPsychol. Behav. 3 (3) (2000) 469–482.	30 healthy OA (mean age = 74.8, SD = 6.18 years old, Range: 65-92)	pre-post (before and after one session of interven-tion protocol)	D: Immersa Desk and Crystal Eyes stereo glasses. I: Immersa Desk			
			C.L. Liu, S.T. Uang, A study of sickness induced within a 3D virtual store and combated with fuzzy control in the elderly, Proc. 9th International Conference on Fuzzy Systems and Knowledge Discovery, IEEE, 2012, pp. 334–338.	32 OA (mean age = 66.5 years) without visual problems	pre-post (before and after one session of interven-tion protocol)	D: 22" stereo-scopic display			

	Virtual Reality Symptom Questionnaire (VRSQ). Test domain: physical and visual effects	This questionnaire assesses eight physical effects: general discomfort, fatigue, boredom, drowsiness, headache, dizziness, concentration difficulties, and nausea, and five visual effects: tired eyes, aching eyes, eyestrain, blurred vision, and difficulties focusing, on a seven-point scale (0–6)	A. Chirico, T. Giovan-netti, P. Neroni, S. Simone, L. Gallo, F. Galli, F. Gian-camilli, M. Predazzi, F. Lucidi, G. De Pietro, et al., Virtual reality for the assessment of everyday cognitive functions in older adults: an evaluation of the virtual reality action test and two interaction devices in a 91-year-old woman, Front. Psychol. 11 (2020).	A female subject of 91 years old independently living	post (after every task in one session of interven-tion protocol)	D: HTC VIVE. I: smart bracelet (Microsoft band 2) and HCT VIVE controllers	yes, online for free, not TUA	https://journals.lww.com/optvissci/FullText/2005/03000/The_Development_of_a_Symptom_Questionnaire_for.8.aspx?casa_token=R1NqlHi-vq8AAAAA:Z6BOmP5dMfxj5XNONM-2NIUGA2ggzozf-zOKjOOuAIbbjxra-HaZ_vFKQA8dVD-X_7hZSlBXJjxQroQxFNmBu5Jrvw8wSo	
			J.P.O. Held, K. Yu, C. Pyles, J.M. Veerbeek, F. Bork, S.M. Heining, N. Navab, A.R. Luft, Augmented reality-based rehabilitation of gait impairments: case report, JMIR MHealth UHealth 8 (5) (2020) e17804.	A man aged 74 years who had a right-hemispheric ischemic stroke	post (after one session of protocol interven-tion)	D: HoloLens 2. I: Xsens system			

(continued)

APPENDIX 1 (Cont'd)

Domain	Questionnaires/ Assestment	Descrption	References	Sample population	Assessment frequency	Technology	Availability		
	Immersive Tendencies Questionnaire (ITQ). Test domains: involvement in common activities and immersive tendencies	This questionnaire measures the capability or tendency of subjects to be involved or immersed, It uses a seven-point scale to measure 29 items f these items that ask for the individual involvement in common activities.	A. Chirico, T. Giovannetti, P. Neroni, S. Simone, L. Gallo, F. Galli, F. Gian-camilli, M. Predazzi, F. Lucidi, G. De Pietro, et al., Virtual reality for the assessment of everyday cognitive functions in older adults: an evaluation of the virtual reality action test and two interaction devices in a 91-year-old woman, Front. Psychol. 11 (2020).	A female subject of 91 years old	post (after one session of protocol intervention)	D: HTC VIVE. I: smart bracelet (Microsoft band 2) and HAT VIVE controllers	yes, online for free, not TUA	file:///C:/Users/mafem/Downloads/ITQ_va.pdf	
			R. Proffitt, B. Lange, C. Chen, C. Winstein, A comparison of older adults' subjective experiences with virtual and real environments during dynamic balance activities, J. Aging Phys. Activ. 23 (1) (2015) 24–33.	30 healthy OA (mean age = 74.37, SD = 8.7, Range: 66–80)	pre (before one session of two task intervention protocol)	D: 32" TV screen. I: PC, MK, ePulse 2™ monitor			

			J.S. McGee, C. van der Zaag, J.G. Buckwalter, M. Thiebaux, A. Van Rooyen, U. Neumann, D. Sisemore, A.A. Rizzo, Issues for the assessment of visuospatial skills in older adults using virtual environment technology, CyberPsychol. Behav. 3 (3) (2000) 469–482.	30 healthy OA (mean age = 74.8, SD = 6.18 years old, Range: 65–92)	pre (before one session of intervention protocol)	D: Immersa Desk and Crystal Eyes stereo glasses. I: Immersa Desk			
Game experience	Game Experience Questionnaire (GEQ). Test domains: During and post game player's feelings and thoughts .	The Game Experience Questionnaire has a modular structure and consists of: 1. The core questionnaire: assesses seven components: Immersion, Flow, Competence, Positive and Negative Affect, Tension,	A. Pyae, T.N. Liukkonen, T. Saarenpaa, M. Luimula, P. Granholm, J. Smed, When Japanese elderly people play a Finnish physical exercise game: a usability study, J. Usability Stud. 11 (4) (2016) 131–152.	21 healthy Finnish OA and 24 healthy Japanese OA (mean age = 84.3, SD = 7.3).	post (after one session of protocol intervention)	D: Tv Screen. I: Xtreme Reality Technology	yes, online for free, not TUA	http://scholar.google.com.co/scholar_url?url=http://www.academia.edu/download/44652437/Game_Experience_Questionnaire_English.doc&hl=es&sa=X&scisig=AAGBfm3AD3BaZLscZJZL6JOx_DjD812EVg&nossl=1&oi=scholarr	

(continued)

APPENDIX 1 (Cont'd)

Domain	Questionnaires/ Assestment	Descrption	References	Sample population	Assessment frequency	Technology	Availability	
		and Challenge 2. The Social Presence Module: measures the empathy, negative Feelings and the behavioural Involvement 3. The Post-game module : measures the Positive Experience, Negative experience, Tiredness, and Returning to Reality components						

			A. Al Mahmud, O. Mubin, S. Shahid, J.B. Martens, Designing social games for children and older adults: two related case studies, Entertain. Comput. 1 (3-4) (2010) 147–156.	8 OA (aged 65–73) CPNR	post (after every task in one session of interve-tion protocol)	D: Projector. I: tangible checkers and camera			
			C., Boletsis, S., McCallum: Augmented reality cubes for cognitive gaming: preliminary usability and game experience testing, International journal of serious games, 3 (1) (2016) 3–18	5 OA (mean age: 67.6, SD: 5.77, range: 61–75) CPNR	post (after 2-month interve-tion protocol at an open and free rate)	D: Tablet, I: AR cubes and Tablet touchpad			
			K. Gerling, P. Dickinson, K. Hicks, L. Mason, A.L. Simeone, K. Spiel, Virtual reality games for people using wheelchairs, Proc. CHI Conference on Human Factors in Computing Systems, 2020 1–11.	16 Adults. Group 1 (mean age = 58, Range: 54 to 65), group 2 (mean age = 82, Range: 67 to 91), both groups with agerelated decrements in motor skills	post (after one session of interven-tion protocol)	D: TV screen, I: WBB			

(continued)

APPENDIX 1 (Cont'd)

Domain	Questionnaires/ Assestment	Descrption	References	Sample population	Assessment frequency	Technology	Availability		
			M. Adcock, F. Sonder, A. Schattin, F. Gennaro, E.D. de Bruin, A usability study of a multicomponent video game-based training for older adults, Eur. Rev. Aging Phys. Activ. 17 (1) (2020) 3.	21 healthy OA (mean age = 71.4, SD = 5.8 years, Range: 65–91)	during-post (after 3 sessions and after a 7 weeks interven- tion protocol, 3 sessions per week)	D: Tv Screen. I: 4 IMUs and PC			
	Core Elements of the Gaming Experience Questionnaire (CEGE). Test domains: Enjoyment, Frustration, Puppetry, Video game, Control, Facilitators, Ownership, Gameplay, and Environment.	This questionnaire has 38 items which are rated using a seven-point Likert scale	Z. Saenz-de Urturi, B. Garc a Zapirain, A. Mendez Zorrilla, Elderly user experience to improve a kinect-based game playability, Behav. Inf. Technol. 34 (11) (2015) 1040–1051.	14 OA (mean age = 81.28, SD = 8.94) with mixed age-related disabilities	each session (3 sessions in 3 different weeks)	D: DC. I: MK	yes, online for free, not TUA	https://www-users.cs.york.ac.uk/~pcairns/pubs/Calvillo_CEGE_2010.pdf	

			A. Chesham, P. Wyss, R.M. Muri, U.P. Mosimann, T. Nef, What older people like to play: genre preferences and acceptance of casual games, JMIR Serious Games 5 (2) (2017) e8.	16 healthy adults aged 65 years and above	post (after one session of interven-tion protocol)	D: 9.7 screen iPad Air 2. I: tablet touchpad			
Physical activ-ity and func-tional fitness	Borg Scale. Test Domains: individual's effort, exertion, breathlessness and fatigue	Measures individual's pain and exertion in a general intensity scale from 0 to 10	R., Kizony, P., Weiss, M., Shahar, D., Rand: Theragame-A Home Based Virtual Reality Rehabilitation System. Esbjerg, Denmark (2006).	12 OA with weak upper extremity (mean age = 70.6, SD = 4.4) 4 OA patients (3 stroke and 1 spinal stenosis)	post (after each task in one session of interven-tion protocol)	D: PC. I: Web cam	yes, online for free, not TUA	https://www.sralab.org/sites/default/files/2018-04/Rating_of_per-ceived_exertion_-_Borg_scale.pdf	sus
			Y. Nagano, K. Ishida, T. Tani, M. Kawasaki, M. Ikeuchi, Short and long-term effects of exergaming for the elderly, Springerplus 5 (1) (2016) 1–10.	42 healthy OA (mean age: 71 ± 5 years , Range: 64–85 years)	initial and final session (2 session per week, 12 weeks of interven-tion protocol)	D: 19-inch display. I: stepping mat that was connected to PC			

(continued)

APPENDIX 1 (Cont'd)

Domain	Questionnaires/ Assestment	Descrption	References	Sample population	Assessment frequency	Technology	Availability	
			T. Okano, D. Kitakoshi, M. Suzuki, A preliminary study on preventive care system based on game playing with communication robots, Proc. Conference on Technologies and Applications of Artificial Intelligence, IEEE, 2013, pp. 84–89.	49 OA (mean age, 71.8 years old) CPNR	post (after one session of interven-tion protocol)	D: Robotic Avatar. I: MK		
			P. Maillot, A. Perrot, A. Hartley, Effects of interactive physical-activity video-game training on physical and cognitive function in older adults, Psychol. Aging 27 (3) (2012) 589.	32 independently OA (Range: 65 and 78 years)	pre (before a interven-tion protocol of 2 sessions per week over a period of 12 weeks)	D: LCD projector. I: Nintendo Wii and WBB		

			L. Taylor, N. Kerse, J. Klenk, R. Borotkanics, R. Maddison, Exergames to improve the mobility of long-term care residents: a cluster randomized controlled trial, Games Health J. 7 (1) (2018) 37–42.	20 OA (mean age = 70.7, SD = 6.4, Range: 65–87) CPNR	post (after each task in one session of interven-tion protocol)	D. TV screen. I: Nintendo Wii, Xbox 360 and MK			
			R. Proffitt, B. Lange, C. Chen, C. Winstein, A comparison of older adults' subjective experiences with virtual and real environments during dynamic balance activities, J. Aging Phys. Activ. 23 (1) (2015) 24–33.	30 healthy OA(mean age = 74.37, SD = 8.7, Range: 66–80)	post (after each task in one session of interven-tion protocol)	D: 32″ TV screen. I: PC, MK, ePulse 2™ monitor			
			M. Adcock, F. Sonder, A. Schattin, F. Gennaro, E.D. de Bruin, A usability study of a multicomponent video game-based training for older adults, Eur. Rev. Aging Phys. Activ. 17 (1) (2020) 3.	21 healthy OA (mean age = 71.4, SD = 5.8 years, Range: 65–91)	each session (after each session in a 7 weeks interven-tion protocol, 3 sessions per week)	D: Tv Screen. I: 4 IMUs and PC			

(continued)

APPENDIX 1 (Cont'd)

Domain	Questionnaires/ Assestment	Descrption	References	Sample population	Assessment frequency	Technology	Availability		
	International Physical Activity Question-naire—Short Form (IPAQ). Test domains: Individual's physical activity	The International Physical Activity Questionnaires (IPAQ) comprises a set of 4 questionnaires that measures physical activity, particularly in large population studies. This questionnaire ask for the time individuals spent being physically active in certain activities in the last 7 days	A.V. Soares, N.B. Junior, M. Hounsell, E. Marcelino, G.M. Rossito, Y.S. Junior, A serious game developed for physical rehabilitation of frail elderly. European research in telemedicine/La Recherche Europ-eenne en, Telemede-cine 5 (2) (2016) 45–53.	24 OA (mean age = 80.9. SD = 5.6 years old) with Frailty syndrome	pre-post (before and after a 10 week interven-tion protocol of 20 sessions, 2 session per week)	D: video projector. I: MK and PC.	yes, online for free, TUA	https://sites.google.com/site/theipaq/	

			R.M. Himmelmeier, R. Nouchi, T. Saito, D. Burin, J. Wiltfang, R. Kawashima, Study protocol: does an acute intervention of high-intensity physical exercise followed by a brain training video game has immediate effects on brain activity of older people during stroop task in FMRI? A randomized controlled trial with crossover design, Front. Aging Neurosci. 11 (2019) 260.	physically active and cognitively healthy OA between 60–70 years old, NPNR	screening (before 4 weeks interven-tion protocol, 1 session per week)	D: Nintendo Dual Screen. I: XL console			
	Senior Fitness Test (SFT). Test domains: indivicual's physical performance	It measures physiologic parameters using functional movement tasks. Test items include: chair stand, arm curl, two minute step test, chair sit and reach, 8-Feet up and go, back scratch test	P. Maillot, A. Perrot, A. Hartley, Effects of interactive physical-activity video-game training on physical and cognitive function in older adults, Psychol. Aging 27 (3) (2012) 589.	32 independently OA (Range: 65 and 78 years)	pre (before a interven-tion protocol of 2 sessions per week over a period of 12 weeks)	D: LCD projector. I: Nintendo Wii and WBB	yes, online for free, TUA	https://www.dnbm.univr.it/documenti/OccorrenzaIns/matdid/matdid182478.pdf	

(continued)

APPENDIX 1 (Cont'd)

Domain	Questionnaires/ Assestment	Descrption	References	Sample population	Assessment frequency	Technology	Availability		
			K. Daniel, Wii-HAB for pre-frail older adults, Rehabil. Nurs. 37 (4) (2012) 195–201.	21 pre-frail OA (mean age = 77, SD = 5.3 years old, Range: 78–80)	pre-post (before and after 15-weeks interven-tion protocol, 21 total sessions)	D: TV screen. I: Nintendo Wii			
			F.R. Sheu, Y.L. Lee, H.T. Hsu, N.S. Chen, Effects of gesture-based fitness games on functional fitness of the elders, Proc. IEEE 15th Interna-tional Conference on Advanced Learning Technologies, IEEE, 2015, pp. 158–160.	10 self-suficient OA (aged 62 to 81)	pre-post (before and after a 4 weeks interven-tion protocol, 3 sessions per week)	D: TV screen. I: Xbox 360 and MK			
			A.R. Goncalves, J.E. Munoz, E.R. Gouveia, M. da Silva Cameirao, S.B. i Badia, Effects of prolonged multidi-mensional fitness training with exergames on the physical exertion levels of older adults, The Visual Computer. (2019) 1–12.	31 active community-dwelling OA (mean age = 67.5, SD = 4.6 years old)	pre (before a 12 weeks interven-tion protocol, 2 session per week)	D: Optoma GT760 projector. I: MK V2, three-axial acceler-ometer ActiGraph WGT3X-BT and PC.			

			B.M. De Queiroz, A.F. Borgatto, A.R. Barbosa, A.V. Guimaraes, Exergame vs. Aerobic exercise and functional fitness of older adults: a randomized controlled trial, J. Phys. Educ. Sport 17 (2) (2017) 740.	36 OA (mean age = 60,25, SD = 3,6 years old, Range: 54–68) reported with depression, anxiety or cardiovascular disease	pre-post (before and after a 12 weeks interven-tion protocol, 3 sessions per week)	D: TV screen. I: Xbox 360 and MK			
	Mini-Balance Evaluation Systems Test (Mini-BES Test). Test Domains: Dynamic balance, anticipatory postural adjustment, reactive postural adjustment, sensory orientation and dynamic gait	It is a 14-item test scored on a 3-level ordinal scale. IT includes 14 items addressing 4 of the 6 sections of the original BESTest.	L. Taylor, N. Kerse, J. Klenk, R. Borotkanics, R. Maddison, Exergames to improve the mobility of long-term care residents: a cluster randomized controlled trial, Games Health J. 7 (1) (2018) 37–42.	20 OA (mean age = 70.7, SD = 6.4, Range: 65–87) CPNR	pre (before one session of interven-tion protocol)	D. TV screen. I: Nintendo Wii, Xbox 360 and MK	yes, online for free, TUA	https://www.sralab.org/sites/default/files/2017-06/MiniBEST_revised_final_3_8_13.pdf	

(continued)

APPENDIX 1 (Cont'd)

Domain	Questionnaires/ Assestment	Descrption	References	Sample population	Assessment frequency	Technology	Availability		
			G.C.V. Gomes, M. do Socorro Simoes, S.M. Lin, J.M.R. Bacha, L.A.P. Viveiro, E.M. Varise, N.C. Junior, B. Lange, W. Jacob Filho, J.E. Pompeu, Feasibility, safety, acceptability, and functional outcomes of playing Nintendo Wii fit PlusTM for frail older adults: a randomized feasibility clinical trial, Maturitas 118 (2018) 20–28.	30 frail and pre-frail OA (mean age = 84, SD = 6, Range 71–92 years old)	pre-post (before and after a 7 weeks interven-tion protocol, 2 sessions per week, and 30 days after the end of the interven-tion)	D: Tv screen. I: Nintendo Wii (Fit Plus)			
			Y. Hutzler, O. Korsensky, Y. Laufer, Rapid stepping test towards virtual visual objects: feasibility and convergent validity in older adults, Technol. Health Care 25 (1) (2017) 49–58.	60 independent OA (mean age = 88.2, SD = 5.0 years old)	pre (before one session of interven-tion protocol)	D: 42-inch TV screen. I: Web cam, MK and PC			

			J.M.R. Bacha, G.C.V. Gomes, T.B. de Freitas, L.A.P. Viveiro, K.G. da Silva, G.C. Bueno, E.M. Varise, C. Torriani-Pasin, A.C. Alonso, N.M.S. Luna, et al., Effects of kinect adventures games versus conventional physical therapy on postural control in elderly people: a randomized controlled trial, Games Health J. 7 (1) (2018) 24–36.	46 OA (mean age 69.3, SD = 5.34 years) capable of walking without assistance, with normal or corrected visual and auditory acuity	pre-post (before and after 7 weeks interven-tios protocol, 2 sessions per week, and 4 weeks after the end of the interven-tion)	D: Tv screen. I: Xbox 360 and MK,			
	Functional Gait Assessment (FGA). Test domains: Postural stability and balance	The FGA is used to assess postural stability during various walking tasks. The individuals are evaluated in 10 items, each item is scored on an ordinal scale from 0–3.	G.C.V. Gomes, M. do Socorro Simoes, S.M. Lin, J.M.R. Bacha, L.A.P. Viveiro, E.M. Varise, N.C. Junior, B. Lange, W. Jacob Filho, J.E. Pompeu, Feasibility, safety, acceptability, and functional outcomes of playing Nintendo Wii fit PlusTM for frail older adults: a randomized feasibility clinical trial, Maturitas 118 (2018) 20–28.	30 frail and pre-frail OA (mean age = 84, SD = 6, Range 71–92 years old)	pre-post (before and after a 7 weeks interven-tion protocol, 2 sessions per week, and 30 days after the end of the interven-tion)	D: Tv screen. I: Nintendo Wii (Fit Plus)	yes, online for free, TUA	https://www.physio-pedia.com/Functional_Gait_Assessment	

(continued)

APPENDIX 1 (Cont'd)

Domain	Questionnaires/ Assestment	Descrption	References	Sample population	Assessment frequency	Technology	Availability		
			J.M.R. Bacha, G.C.V. Gomes, T.B. de Freitas, L.A.P. Viveiro, K.G. da Silva, G.C. Bueno, E.M. Varise, C. Torriani-Pasin, A.C. Alonso, N.M.S. Luna, et al., Effects of kinect adventures games versus conventional physical therapy on postural control in elderly people: a randomized controlled trial, Games Health J. 7 (1) (2018) 24–36.	46 OA (mean age 69.3, SD = 5.34 years) capable of walking without assistance, with normal or corrected visual and auditory acuity	pre-post (before and after 7 weeks interven-tios protocol, 2 sessions per week, and 4 weeks after the end of the interven-tion)	D: Tv screen. I: Xbox 360 and MK,			
	Berg Balance scale. Test domains: Static balance and fall risk.	It is a 14 item list consisting of a five-point scale ranging from 0 to 4. This scale determines a subject ability to safely balance during a series of predetermined tasks.	J.K. Dal Jae Im, Y.J. Kim, S. Cho, Y.K. Cho, T. Lim, H.S. Lee, H.J. Kim, Y.J. Kang, Utility of a three-dimensional interactive augmented reality program for balance and mobility rehabilitation in the elderly: a feasibility study, Ann. Rehabil. Med. 39 (3) (2015) 462.	18 community-dwell-ing OA (mean age = 64.70, SD = 7.27, Range: 56–76 years) walking independently	pre-post (before and after a 4 weeks interven-tion protocol, 10 total sessions)	D: LSD screen. I: Xbox 360, MK and PC	yes, online for free, TUA	https://www.physio-pedia.com/Berg_Balance_Scale	

			N. Katajapuu, M. Luimula, Y.L. Theng, T.P. Pham, J. Li, A. Pyae, K. Sato, Benefits of exergame exercise on physical functioning of elderly people, Proc. 8th IEEE International Conference on Cognitive Infocommunications (CogInfoCom), IEEE, 2017, pp. 000085–000090.	30 OA (Mean age = 71.34, SD = 6.62) with neurological status or some kind of a cognitive/mental disorder	pre-post (before and after 6 weeks intervention protocol, 2 sessions per week)	D: PC. I: MK			
			K.H. Cho, K.J. Lee, C.H. Song, Virtual-reality balance training with a video-game system improves dynamic balance in chronic stroke patients, Tohoku J. Exp. Med. 228 (1) (2012) 69–74.	22 OA (63,26 years old) stroke patients	pre-post (before and after 6 weeks intervention protocol, 3 sessions per week)	D:42-inch LCD screen. I:WBB			

(continued)

APPENDIX 1 (Cont'd)

Domain	Questionnaires/ Assestment	Descrption	References	Sample population	Assessment frequency	Technology	Availability	
	Timed Up and Go Test (TUG). Test domains: Mobility and balance impairments	The TUG test requires scores the time that a subject takes to rise from a chair, walk 3.0 m at a comfortable pace to a mark placed on the floor, turn around at the 3.0 m mark, walk back to the starting point, and return to sitting in the chair.	Y. Hutzler, O. Korsensky, Y. Laufer, Rapid stepping test towards virtual visual objects: feasibility and convergent validity in older adults, Technol. Health Care 25 (1) (2017) 49–58.	60 independent OA (mean age = 88.2, SD = 5.0 years old)	pre (before one session of interven-tion protocol)	D: 42-inch TV screen. I: Web cam, MK and PC	yes, online for free, TUA	https://www.thompsonhealth.com/Portals/0/_RehabilitationServices/PT%20Mgmt%20of%20Knee/Functional_Tests.pdf
			A.V. Soares, N.B. Junior, M. Hounsell, E. Marcelino, G.M. Rossito, Y.S. Junior, A serious game developed for physical rehabilitation of frail elderly. European research in telemedicine/La Recherche Europ-eenne en, Telemede-cine 5 (2) (2016) 45–53.	24 OA (mean age = 80.9. SD = 5.6 years old) with Frailty syndrome	pre-post (before and after a 10 week interven-tion protocol of 20 sessions, 2 session per week)	D: video projector. I: MK and PC.		

			E.C. Park, S.G. Kim, C.W. Lee, The effects of virtual reality game exercise on balance and gait of the elderly, J. Phys. Ther. Sci. 27 (4) (2015) 1157–1159.	30 OA (mean age = 66.5, SD = 8.1 year old, Range: > 65 years old)	pre-post	D: Tv screen. I: Nintendo Wii and WBB			
			T.E. Shubert, J. Basnett, A. Chokshi, M. Barrett, R. Komatireddy, Are virtual rehabilitation technologies feasible models to scale an evidence-based fall prevention program? A pilot study using the kinect camera, JMIR Rehabil. Assist. Technol. 2 (2) (2015) e10.	21 OA (mean age = 69.2, SD = 5.8) with mixed chronic diseases (no neurodegenerative)	pre (before a a 90-minute session of interven-tion protocol)	D: PC, I: MK			
			J.K. Dal Jae Im, Y.J. Kim, S. Cho, Y.K. Cho, T. Lim, H.S. Lee, H.J. Kim, Y.J. Kang, Utility of a three-dimensional interactive augmented reality program for balance and mobility rehabilitation in the elderly: a feasibility study, Ann. Rehabil. Med. 39 (3) (2015) 462.	18 community-dwell-ing OA (mean age = 64.70, SD = 7.27, Range: 56–76 years) walking independently	pre-post (before and after a 4 weeks interven-tion protocol, 10 total sessions)	D: LSD screen. I: Xbox 360, MK and PC			

(continued)

APPENDIX 1 (Cont'd)

Domain	Questionnaires/ Assestment	Descrption	References	Sample population	Assessment frequency	Technology	Availability		
			K.H. Cho, K.J. Lee, C.H. Song, Virtual-reality balance training with a video-game system improves dynamic balance in chronic stroke patients, Tohoku J. Exp. Med. 228 (1) (2012) 69–74.	22 OA (63,26 years old) stroke patients	pre-post (before and after 6 weeks interven-tion protocol, 3 sessions per week)	D: 42-inch LCD screen. I: WBB			
			Y. Nagano, K. Ishida, T. Tani, M. Kawasaki, M. Ikeuchi, Short and long-term effects of exergaming for the elderly, Springerplus 5 (1) (2016) 1–10.	42 healthy OA (mean age: 71 ± 5 years, Range: 64–85 years)	pre-post (before and after 2 session per week, 12 weeks of interven-tion protocol)	D: 19-inch display. I: stepping mat that was connected to PC			
			L. Taylor, N. Kerse, J. Klenk, R. Borotkanics, R. Maddison, Exergames to improve the mobility of long-term care residents: a cluster randomized controlled trial, Games Health J. 7 (1) (2018) 37–42.	20 OA (mean age = 70.7, SD = 6.4, Range: 65–87) CPNR	pre (before one session of interven-tion protocol)	D. TV screen. I: Nintendo Wii, Xbox 360 and MK			

Cognitive assessment	Mini-Mental State Examination (MMSE). Test domains: orientation, attention, calculation, recall, language and motor skills.	The MMSE offers a quick and simple way to quantify cognitive function and screen for cognitive loss.	J. Gerlowska, U. Skrobas, K. Grabowska-Aleksandrowicz, A. Korchut, S. Szklener, D. Szczesniak-Stanczyk, D. Tzovaras, K. Rejdak, Assessment of perceived attractiveness, usability, and societal impact of a multimodal robotic assistant for aging patients with memory impairments, Front. Neurol. 9 (2018) 392.	10 OA and 8 OAwith mild cognitive impairments (MCI) (Range 60–81 years old)	screening	D: Tablet. I: Robotic assistant prototype	yes, online for free, TUA	https://www.bgs.org.uk/sites/default/files/content/attachment/2018-07-05/mini-mental_state_exam.pdf	
			G. Corno, S. Bouchard, H. Forget, Usability assessment of the virtual multitasking test (V-MT) for elderly people, Annu. Rev. Cyberther. Telemed. 199 (2014) 168–172.	10 OA (age > 60) without any diagnosis of cognitive impairment.	screening (before one session of intervention protocol)	D: CAVE, HMD. IHMD controllers			
			Z. Saenz-de Urturi, B. Garc a Zapirain, A. Mendez Zorrilla, Elderly user experience to improve a kinect-based game playability, Behav. Inf. Technol. 34 (11) (2015) 1040–1051.	14 OA (mean age = 81.28, SD = 8.94) with mixed age-related disabilities	pre (before an intervention protocol pf 3 sessions in 3 different weeks)	D: DC. I: MK			

(continued)

APPENDIX 1 (Cont'd)

Domain	Questionnaires/ Assestment	Descrption	References	Sample population	Assessment frequency	Technology	Availability		
			H. Fordell, K. Bodin, G. Bucht, J. Malm, A virtual reality test battery for assessment and screening of spatial neglect, Acta Neurol. Scand. 123 (3) (2011) 167–174.	31 OA (mean = 74,1, SD = 11 years old), post-stroke patients	screening (before one session of interven-tion protocol)	D: 19 CRT monitor and shutter glasses. I: DC, head-phones, robotic pen and keyboard.			
			K.H. Cho, K.J. Lee, C.H. Song, Virtual-reality balance training with a video-game system improves dynamic balance in chronic stroke patients, Tohoku J. Exp. Med. 228 (1) (2012) 69–74.	22 OA (63,26 years old) stroke patients	screening (before 6 weeks interven-tion protocol, 3 sessions per week)	D: 42-inch LCD screen. I: WBB			
			A.V. Soares, N.B. Junior, M. Hounsell, E. Marcelino, G.M. Rossito, Y.S. Junior, A serious game developed for physical rehabilitation of frail elderly. European research in telemedicine/La Recherche Europ-eenne en, Telemede-cine 5 (2) (2016) 45–53.	24 OA (mean age = 80.9. SD = 5.6 years old) with Frailty syndrome	pre-post (before and after a 10 week interven-tion protocol of 20 sessions, 2 session per week)	D: video projector. I: MK and PC.			

			R.M. Himmelmeier, R. Nouchi, T. Saito, D. Burin, J. Wiltfang, R. Kawashima, Study protocol: does an acute intervention of high-intensity physical exercise followed by a brain training video game has immediate effects on brain activity of older people during stroop task in FMRI? A randomized controlled trial with crossover design, Front. Aging Neurosci. 11 (2019) 260.	physically active and cognitively healthy OA between 60-70 years old, NPNR	screening (before 4 weeks interven- tion protocol, 1 session per week)	D: Nintendo Dual Screen. I: XL console		
			A.R. Goncalves, J.E. Munoz, E.R. Gouveia, M. da Silva Cameirao, S.B. i Badia, Effects of prolonged multidi- mensional fitness training with exergames on the physical exertion levels of older adults, Vis. Comput. (2019) 1–12.	31 active community- dwelling OA (mean age = 67.5, SD = 4.6 years old)	screening (before a 12 weeks interven- tion protocol, 2 session per week)	D: Optoma GT760 projector. I: MK V2, three-axial acceler- ometer ActiGraph WGT3X- BT and PC.		

(continued)

APPENDIX 1 (Cont'd)

Domain	Questionnaires/ Assestment	Descrption	References	Sample population	Assessment frequency	Technology	Availability		
			J.K. Dal Jae Im, Y.J. Kim, S. Cho, Y.K. Cho, T. Lim, H.S. Lee, H.J. Kim, Y.J. Kang, Utility of a three-dimensional interactive augmented reality program for balance and mobility rehabilitation in the elderly: a feasibility study, Ann. Rehabil. Med. 39 (3) (2015) 462.	18 community-dwelling OA (mean age = 64.70, SD = 7.27, Range: 56–76 years) walking independently	pre (before a 4 weeks intervention protocol, 10 total sessions)	D: LSD screen. I: Xbox 360, MK and PC.			
	Montreal Cognitive Assessment (MoCA). Test domains: attention and concentration, executive functions, memory, language, visuoconstructional skills, conceptual thinking, calculations, and orientation	Is a 30 point test used as rapid screening instrument for mild cognitive dysfunction.	B. Keshavarz, R. Ramkhalawansingh, B. Haycock, S. Shahab, J. Campos, Comparing simulator sickness in younger and older adults during simulated driving under different multisensory conditions, Transp. Res. F Traffic Psychol. Behav. 54 (2018) 47–62.	58 YA (aged 18–35) and 63 OA (age 65+), normal state of health	screening (before one session of intervention protocol)	D: digital speedometer displayed and Samsung Galaxy tablet. I: Logitech G27 steering wheel, gas and brake pedals, and Samsung Galaxy tablet touchpad	yes, online for free, TUA	https://www.parkinsons.va.gov/resources/MOCA-Test-English.pdf	

			T. Vanbellingen, S.J. Filius, T. Ny eler, E.E. van Wegen, Usability of videogame-based dexterity training in the early rehabilitation phase of stroke patients: a pilot study, Front. Neurol. 8 (2017) 654.	13 OA (mean age = 68.2, SD = 17.5) post-stroke patients	screening (before a intervention protocol of 9 sessions of 30 min, 3 times per week)	D: DC. I: Leap Motion Controller			
			J.M.R. Bacha, G.C.V. Gomes, T.B. de Freitas, L.A.P. Viveiro, K.G. da Silva, G.C. Bueno, E.M. Varise, C. Torriani-Pasin, A.C. Alonso, N.M.S. Luna, et al., Effects of kinect adventures games versus conventional physical therapy on postural control in elderly people: a randomized controlled trial, Games Health J. 7 (1) (2018) 24–36.	46 OA (mean age 69.3, SD = 5.34 years) capable of walking without assistance, with normal or corrected visual and auditory acuity	pre-post (before and after 7 weeks interventios protocol, 2 sessions per week, and 4 weeks after the end of the intervention)	D: Tv screen. I: Xbox360 and MK			

(continued)

APPENDIX 1 (Cont'd)

Domain	Questionnaires/ Assestment	Descrption	References	Sample population	Assessment frequency	Technology	Availability	
			G.C.V. Gomes, M. do Socorro Simoes, S.M. Lin, J.M.R. Bacha, L.A.P. Viveiro, E.M. Varise, N.C. Junior, B. Lange, W. Jacob Filho, J.E. Pompeu, Feasibility, safety, acceptability, and functional outcomes of playing Nintendo Wii fit PlusTM for frail older adults: a randomized feasibility clinical trial, Maturitas 118 (2018) 20–28.	30 frail and pre-frail OA (mean age = 84, SD = 6, Range 71–92 years old)	pre-post (before and after a 7 weeks interven-tion protocol, 2 sessions per week, and 30 days after the end of the interven-tion)	D: Tv screen. I: Nintendo Wii (Fit Plus)		
			H. Huygelier, B. Schraepen, R. van Ee, V.V. Abeele, C.R. Gillebert, Acceptance of immersive head-mounted virtual reality in older adults, Sci. Rep. 9 (1) (2019) 1–12.	72 OA (mean age = 74.8, SD = 10.4, Range: 60–92) CPNR	post (after one session of protocol interven-tion)	D: Oculus Rift HMD, I: Oculus Rift controllers and PC		

Abbreviations: AR: augmented Reality, CPNR: Condition of population not reported. D:Display, DC: Desktop Computer, HDM: Head Mounted Display, I: Interface, NPNR: number of participants not reported, MK: Microsoft Kinect, OA: older adults PC: personal computer, pre: previous to protocol, pre-post: previous and posterior to protocol, post: posterior to protocol, SD: standard deviation, TUA: training to use the assessment, WBB: Wii Balance Board, YA: Young adults.

TABLE 7.1 Summary of questionnaires/assessments often used with serious games for older adults.

Domain	Questionnaires/assessment	References	Sample population	Assessment frequency
Usability	System usability scale: Test domain: perceived usability	[78, 84, 23, 13, 97, 114, 2, 70, 113]	Healthy OA and OA with mixed age-related disabilities or post stroke (age range: 59–91)	Post
	Ad-hoc usability questionnaire (created by the authors based on previous usability test)	[88, 32, 30]	Healthy OA and OA post stroke (age range: 60–85)	During and post
	User experience questionnaire. Test domains: efficiency, perspicuity, dependability, originality, and stimulation.	[29, 60, 34]	Healthy OA and OA with atrial fibrillation (age range: 60–87)	Post
Virtual reality	Simulator sickness questionnaire. Test domains: nausea, oculomotor, and disorientation	[23, 44, 58, 49, 65]	Healthy older adults (age range: 60–92)	Pre and Post
	Virtual reality symptom questionnaire. Test domain: physical and visual effects	[20, 40]	Healthy OA and OA post stroke (age range: 74–91)	Post
	Immersive tendencies questionnaire. Test domains: involvement in common activities and immersive tendencies	[20, 65, 89]	Healthy OA (age range: 65–92)	Pre and Post
Game experience	Game experience questionnaire. Test domains: During and postgame player's feelings and thoughts.	[90, 3, 13, 33,2]	Healthy OA and OA with age-related decrements in motor skills (age range: 61–94)	Post
	Core elements of the gaming experience questionnaire. Test domains: enjoyment, frustration, puppetry, video game, control, facilitators, ownership, gameplay, and environment.	[113, 19]	Healthy OA and OA with mixed age-related disabilities (age range: 65–90)	Each session and post

(continued)

TABLE 7.1 (Cont'd)

Domain	Questionnaires/assessment	References	Sample population	Assessment frequency
Physical activity and functional fitness	Borg Scale. Test Domains: individual's effort, exertion, breathlessness, and fatigue	[50, 75, 79, 61, 107, 89, 2]	Healthy OA and OA with weak upper extremity (age range: 65–90)	Screening, pre and post
	International physical activity questionnaire. Test domains: Individual's physical activity	[102, 41]	Healthy OA and OA with frailty syndrome (age range: 60–86)	Each session, pre and post
	Senior fitness test (SFT). Test domains: individual's physical performance	[61, 26, 96, 36, 27]	Healthy OA and OA reported with depression, anxiety or cardiovascular disease, and OA frail and prefrail (age range: 60–86)	Pre and Post
	Mini-Balance Evaluation Systems Test (Mini-BESTest). Test Domains: Dynamic balance, anticipatory postural adjustment, reactive postural adjustment, sensory orientation, and dynamic gait	107, 35, 43,8]	Healthy OA and OA frail and prefrail (age range: 58–92)	Pre and Post
	Functional Gait Assessment. Test domains: Postural stability and balance	[35, 8]	Healthy OA and OA frail and pre-frail (age range: 71–92)	Pre and Post
	Berg balance scale. Test domains: Static balance and fall risk.	[25, 47, 21]	Healthy OA and OA with neurological status or some kind of a cognitive/mental disorder, and OA post stroke (age range: 56–78)	Pre and Post
	Timed Up and Go Test (TUG). Test domains: Mobility and balance impairments	[43, 102, 81, 97, 25, 21, 75, 107]	Healthy OA, OA with mixed chronic diseases, and OA post stroke (age range: 58–87)	Pre and Post
Cognitive assessment	Mini-Mental State Examination (MMSE). Test domains: orientation, attention, calculation, recall, language, and motor skills.	[34, 23, 113, 32, 21, 102, 41, 36, 25]	Healthy OA, OA with mild cognitive impairments, OA mixed age-related disabilities, OA with frailty syndrome and OA post stroke (age range: 56–86)	Screening, pre and post
	Montreal Cognitive Assessment (MoCA). Test domains: attention and concentration, executive functions, memory, language, visuoconstructional skills, conceptual thinking, calculations, and orientation	[49, 114, 8, 35, 44]	Healthy OA, frail and prefrail OA, and OA post stroke (age range: 51–92)	Screening, pre and post

Abbreviations: OA: older adults, Pre: previous to protocol, Pre-post: previous and posterior to protocol, Post: posterior to protocol.

7.5 Application areas and tools

7.5.1 Application domains

Several taxonomies have been proposed to better categorize the different serious games for health. For instance, a taxonomy that describes the different modalities for exergames (e.g., competitive vs noncompetitive) proposed the inclusion of social aspects such as collaboration and players' involvement [71]. Games created for rehabilitation purposes have been categorized considering important application areas (e.g., cognitive, physical, behavioral) as well as application subareas (e.g., upper limb rehabilitation or working memory training) and targeted populations (e.g., people living with dementia [64]). Following the taxonomy proposed by Sawyer and Smith [94] and considering games for health that are popularly used by older adults, we have extracted three important categories: (1) preventative, (2) therapeutic, and (3) assessment.

7.5.1.1 Preventative

Serious games that promote physical activity and mental training to improve abilities with the intention of mitigating risk of an undesired event occurring (e.g., improving cardiovascular health to reduce the risk of heart disease) are categorized as *preventive*. Some content developed for commercially available exergaming consoles (e.g., Wii, Kinect) to promote health have been negatively received by older adults, which is why the recent games include specific design issues for this population [15].

Preventative interventions need to focus on longer term engagement and regular use. This is often accomplished using multiple gaming elements (challenges, points, rewards, mechanics) [74] to help align actions better with older adults' abilities and changes in these abilities over time, encouraging physical activity in a way that allows for easier repetition in true-to-life scenarios [46]. This is one of the reasons why games that simulate traditional sports and daily activities are particularity well received by older adults. The promotion of physical activity through games has also been shown to result in increased confidence in older adults' use of technology, which has the potential of supporting increased engagement in other areas of their life. For example, technological proficiency can improve connectedness with family and friends, enable greater access to information and programs of interest, and support positive self-image [46].

Games for mental training have been shown to attenuate cognitive decline in aging for some populations [9, 61]. However, the research community is still seeking evidence of transference of cognitive training in one domain to other cognitive domains and activities of daily living in older adults [10, 119].

7.5.1.2 *Therapeutic*

Therapeutic serious games are usually developed with rehabilitation as their main goal. Games and VR are an attractive approach as they can provide new tools to perform therapeutic tasks in an engaging manner that can motivate patients who would otherwise lack interest or motivation to complete them [7]. Most of these games are intended to be a complement of traditional rehabilitation therapies as there is still a lack of evidence of advantages over the conventional methods [69]. Therapeutic games for older adults are often centered on improving movement (joint range of movement and balance) [25, 8] and cognitive features (spatial orientation, sustained attention, and memory) [88, 5, 9] that can be used in older adults with stroke, dementia, or Parkinson's disease.

7.5.1.3 *Assessment*

The use of serious games to detect symptoms or to assess people with physical or cognitive impairments has been proposed as an objective and complementary method to the traditional measurements, which usually use scales and questionnaires. The assessment is focused on the digitization, storing, and processing of game events that can be captured during the interaction, such as spatial orientation [32] or balance and gait [67], which are present in the detection of neurodegenerative disorders such as dementia of Alzheimer's type and other dementias [22, 111], mild cognitive impairment, and Parkinson's disease [6, 67]. In these approaches, the assessment is often automatically extracted from gameplay performance. Reliable and accurate assessment is beneficial from the perspective of the clinician and patient as it is can be less stressful and less degrading than taking a standardized assessment. It can also be repeated relatively consistently over time through multiple gameplay opportunities.

Many of these games use immersive technologies (such as VR) due that the vividness of the content and the interactivity of the tasks. These appear to have advantages for ecological cognitive assessment and rehabilitation [67, 24]. Researchers have explored serious games mainly for the assessment of body movement to monitor and understand sensorimotor recovery. This monitoring is useful to detect the improvement of physical rehabilitation after injuries or stroke, searching for patterns in the movement reflected in metrics that measure joint angles [95]. Physiological metrics have been proposed in games that use human body signals [36, 8] to look at objective measurements of improvement in cardiovascular regulation. The assessment of cognitive skills has been explored, such as the development of a virtual game as a screening tool for cognitive health (e.g., MoCA) [13]. The work of Jung et al. [45] describes a game to estimate specific cognitive functions as they appear in the MMSE test. Novel VR games for memory assessment have been developed [88] to try and replace/complement traditional paper-and-pencil measures for spatial memory in cognitive tasks [83]. Finally, researchers have proposed the use of VR-based driving assessment systems to be used as interactive tools to overcome limitations of conventional assessments (e.g., subjective interpretation, variance of the procedures) [128].

7.5.2 Available software/hardware tools for technology adoption

7.5.2.1 Software and visual assets

Gaming technologies are constantly evolving and this represents a challenge for researchers as keeping up with this development pace carries several complex steps. While research into serious games should consider innovative, cutting edge, and scientifically significant approaches, the field often fails in creating technologies that are more sustainable, agile, and effective for rapid and successful uptake to the consumer market [48]. Without this, many of the excellent advances made in research become obsolete before they can be implemented and assessed through widespread uptake by older adults and other end-users. A critical aspect to facilitate the rapid adoption of technology for supporting older adults is the design, development, and free distribution (e.g., open source) of interactive tools that have been specifically crated for older adults. Efforts toward creating and making available software tools that can aid the multistage process of creating specialized games for older adults have been published in the last decade [105, 72, 77]. Some of the most important tools allowing agile and flexible prototyping and testing can be grouped as follows:

- *Tools for rapid content design and development:* The creation of novel gaming tools for older adults should be a highly iterative, multistage, and integrative process that requires expertise such as 3D modeling, game design, and programming. Some of the available tools that have been created and piloted to streamline the process of prototyping games and virtual content targeting older adults are: (1) NeuroVR tool [92], a cost-free software tool that provides a game editor for the creation/modification of virtual environments, (2) Reha@Panel [116], an open and distributed (across multiple tools) architecture for motor and neurorehabilitation "in-home" using interactive tools and, (3) FAAST [119], a middleware (tool that bridges gaps between applications) that facilitates full-body control with games using the Kinect sensor.
- *Assets for content creation:* Researchers in the fields of serious game design, technology for aging, and gerontology have been investigating the feasibility of using different software tools for content creation as well as the specific virtual elements that are

appealing for older adults. A set of freely available, standardized, and validated 3D household objects for VR therapy and research has been proposed to aid recognizability, familiarity, and visual complexity in immersive applications targeting older adults [108]. Furthermore, older player's archetypes and willingness to use exergames for physical activity promotion were investigated in a project aiming to facilitate the use of UCD tools for exergame design targeting older adults [74].

- *Accessible, age-friendly gaming content:* Two initiatives stand out for enabling free access of the serious games after research trials have ended: (1) Open Rehab Initiative (https://openrehab.org/) that allows access to games and other tools previously used in geriatric rehabilitation and (2) Wii habilitation (http://www.wiihabilitation.co.uk/) that publishes content on how to use commercially available consoles and games (e.g., Kinect, Wii) and adapt them for older adults. Beyond these research-based networks, the fitness gaming portal (https://www.fitness-gaming.com/) has a comprehensive and updated list of companies that offer products and services that can be purchased by healthcare institutions looking to adopt a developed solution.
- *Interactive assessment tools:* Tools for evaluating physical fitness aspects in older adults using gaming systems and interfaces have been designed using multiple hardware tools (e.g., custom-made multisensor platforms [110] and low-cost depth cameras [37]). Commercially available systems such as the Wii Balance Board have been used to evaluate posture and postural control in poststroke participants [59]. Other interactive tools have been used to assess important cognitive functionalities of older adults such as executive functions and language [31] as well as specific elements of the memory (e.g., episodic memory [87]). The potential of game-based metrics to model older adult's mental health is rapidly gaining attraction as a method to capture important aging-related parameters that can be potentially used as biomarkers [62]. This is a key factor in enabling the comparison and improvement of available approaches.

7.5.2.2 Hardware and interfaces

- *Display modalities*: For VR technologies, the hardware can be divided into nonimmersive, semi-immersive, and fully immersive systems. Nonimmersive systems or "conventional systems" are lower interaction single-monitor or small 2D screens (e.g., desktop computer, laptop computer, tablet, smartphone). An alternative to conventional 2D screen is the projection, which is present in large white screens or walls, and sometimes is preferred because it allows a large interactive play area. Semi-immersive systems can be seen as large monitors/projectors that elicit greater feelings of being physically present than that of conventional screens. Immersive systems enable a high degree of visual immersion characterized by the use of tools such as a head-mounted display (HMDs) or surrounded projections (e.g., Cave Automatic Virtual Environments, CAVEs). The increasing availability, both in terms of pervasiveness and cost, of these technologies has enabled the spread of their use in all kinds of communities ranging from entertainment and training to education and rehabilitation [112].

As with all user types, it is important to consider older adults' lived experience to create complementary interventions. Most older adults are most familiar with a TV screen as the primary screen-based medium, although familiarity with computers and smartphones rapidly increasing. This is why the nonimmersive systems, such as a conventional 2D screen, are the main display used in several studies for this population; it is a relatively familiar technology that is less of a cognitive challenge to understand [112]. Complementing their increasing uptake and day-to-day use by older adults, smartphones, computers, and tablets are being developed as well [85]. Researchers have used phones and tablets to implement simple games for cognitive and physical training [85, 78], monitor the general health status of older adults [60], and support medication management [29].

With respect to immersive hardware, HMDs are the most popular for displaying virtual content and because of their relative accessibility and decreasing costs. Preliminary studies on the use of HMD's attractiveness for older adults have shown that their attitudes toward this type of technology can vary. While many may be skeptical, studies such as [44] demonstrated positive changes in attitudes toward immersive VR after the first exposure in a group of 76 healthy older adults. However, HMDs can induce cybersickness symptoms and lead to low cognitive performance of participants; this is especially not well studied yet for older adult users and must be considered in their development [88, 23]. CAVE systems, which use multiple projections on the walls and floor that surrounds the user, seem to cause less motion-sickness, improve presence and agency, and are becoming less expensive [36].

In general, despite minor interaction issues and errors in interaction, virtual systems are rated as usable and feasible by older adults [112]. Moreover, these technologies have shown positive effects on older adults' social and emotional wellbeing and importantly the participants reported being satisfied with the technology [38].

- *Input interfaces*: Another important aspect that drives the development of interactive technologies to support aging is the interface (i.e., what enables users to communicate with games). Most of the systems currently on the market are not designed to accommodate for older adults' physical and cognitive abilities or limitations [38]. Older adults may be slower in learning new technologies (compared with younger populations) or may respond better to instructions that are given in a different way. As with all users, older adults are more likely to have feelings of low self-efficacy, anxiety, and hostility when such technologies are difficult to understand and use [39]; namely, the technology is not meeting their needs. Therefore, natural (e.g., intuitive-to-use) input devices are required to create immersive, engaging, and truly interactive experiences.

Mobile phones and tablet interactions are performed through touch-pads, which sometimes are not intuitive for older adults or are difficult to use because of reduced eyesight, reduced dexterity, and greater prevalence of tremors [103]. The classic interfaces used for games are the hand-held motion controllers (e.g., gamepads, joysticks). Research has shown that this is not an optimal interface for older adults, who have reported usability issues with joysticks and VR controllers due to the complexity of button combinations [23, 112]. Simple modifications of the joystick could facilitate their use with older adults. Commercially available joysticks for users with special needs (e.g., Xbox Adaptive Controller) have been explored to varying degrees of success [51]. More advanced exergaming technologies have included motion sensors (e.g., inertial motor units) that can track human movements precisely. Wii's tracker technology makes the controllers intuitive to use, which results in easier and greater adaptation by older adults to play exergames [57]. Some of these motion-tracking technologies can be found in wearable sensors; however previous studies have shown that older adults find them more invasive and unpleasant than ambient sensors that are placed in the environment [38]. Along this approach, computer vision technologies such as the camera-based tracking systems (e.g., Kinect sensor) have the advantage of being less intrusive, capture more information, and allow free movement of the user being tracked [51]. However, older adults have different perceptions regarding these systems with some agreeing with the user-friendly benefit, while others had difficulties, such as learning how to use gesture controls and navigating the menus using "air gestures" [39, 63].

Differences in attitudes are in part because of the perceived complexity of the interface. Step platforms, such as Wii balance board (no air gestures or buttons are required), have been used as an alternative input interface, mostly use for balance and postural rehabilitation with no reported difficulty in the use of the system [81, 61, 21]. Other interesting interface that can be used to facilitate the interaction with games by older adults is exercise equipment. While connectivity to stationary bikes and treadmills as exergame input interfaces is increasing (Nintendo has even created their own interface called cyberbike), relatively little has been done to understand their potential for older adults [4]. For example, Pedroli et al.[84] tested a cycle-ergonometer in immersive setups (e.g., CAVE environments) to promote physical activity; however, the majority of such systems have been not explored with older adults [82, 98]. Following the approach of using already existing equipment as interface, wheelchairs have been explored as interface in VR prototypes created with people with mobility impairments.

In summary, while there are many ways serious games can be developed to support a diversity of older adult needs and trends in useful applications are emerging, the appropriate design and use of software, hardware, and interfaces is under-explored and requires greater systematic research.

7.6 Adaptive serious gaming systems

Older adults tend to have a greater range of abilities than younger ones. Moreover, these abilities are often dynamic in nature. Thus, the ability of these systems to deliver a personalized and reconfigurable experience would support their broader applicability. That said, an increase in complexity will deter use by older adults and other primary users (e.g., rehabilitation therapists). The creation of *adaptive serious gaming systems* that are more intelligent, aware of, and complementary to multiple aspects of the interaction of the older adult with the system could support greater engagement and efficacy.

One approach to considering adaptive systems are the four categories put forward by Hou et al. [42], which defines dynamic changes of the player/operator's state that can elicit important data to drive automatic adaptations: (1) behavioral: what the player is doing, (2) physiological: internal state of body and mind, (3) contextual: inference based on surroundings or working environment, and (4) subjective: what the player communicates about his/her own state. An adaptive layer (see Fig. 7.1) can be thought of as a software entity empowered with system intelligent algorithms that processes various inputs to create adaptations (offline or online/real-time) that semi-autonomously or autonomously deliver a more enjoyable, effective, and highly-personalized game experience. As explained in Section 7.2, information can be displayed in multiple devices ranging from conventional 2D screens, large displays (e.g., projections), or immersive displays such as HMD-VRs. The displayed information is useful in enabling players to create adaptations and modify their behavior to achieve their desired state (e.g., specific range of motion, desired level of perceived exertion). Examples of adaptive exergaming that uses heart rate information to enhance cardiorespiratory training in older adults have shown players can spend up to 40% more time in their target zones

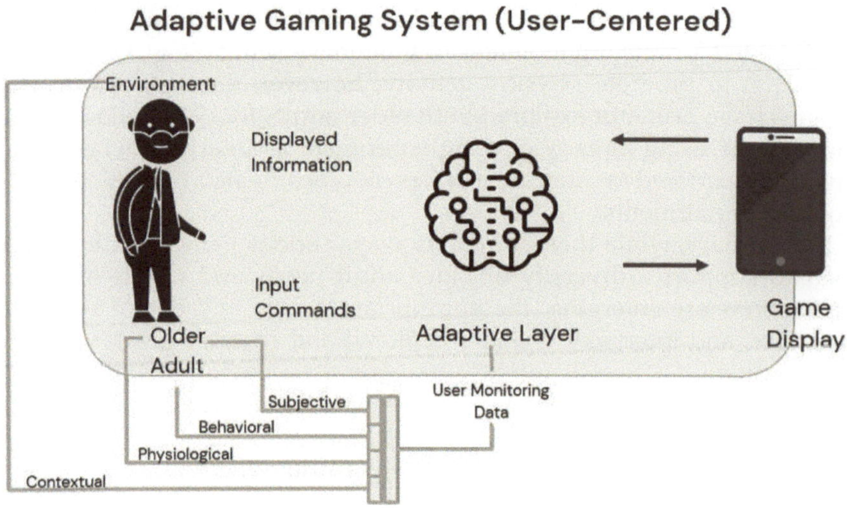

FIG. 7.1 Overview of a user-centered adaptive gaming system.

compared to the conventional exercises [72]. Other adaptive modalities have been proposed including, but not limited to, the use neurophysiological data, for instance, the use of surface electroencephalography to self-control neural rhythms and the feedback of Electromyography signal to control robotic sensors [68]; or kinematic information [73] to dynamically personalized game experience and goals. Adapting serious games used in healthcare applications involving older adults should take a holistic approach that can use data (often from multiple sources) and interpret them to create more informed, contextualized, reactive, and personalized gaming systems.

Despite progress in system intelligence and machine learning algorithms, more research is needed to better understand the role of adaptive systems to boost the effectiveness of serious games for health. This is particularity important for vulnerable populations that often have optimal exercise target zones that are nonhomogeneous and dynamic; indeed, some have limits that can be harmful to their health if they are exceeded (e.g., older adults who are using beta blockers to help regulate their blood pressure). Therefore, adaptive systems, particularly fully autonomous ones, must be designed and tested carefully to ensure they are working with what is best for each individual to positively support the users' needs. While this is a major challenge, more research is needed to create adaptive systems that can run across platforms and technologies (e.g., HMDs, mobile phones) and have the capability to be integrated in different virtual contents (e.g., physiological adaptation [72]).

7.7 Challenges and opportunities in VR and exergaming research

The field serious gaming has been growing and consolidating its scientific evidence as an effective addition to promoting a healthy lifestyle for older adults. Despite all the positive benefits and the enthusiasm of the research community, research into serious gaming is still is in its infancy with several challenges that must be overcome before becoming truly accessible and effective. These include the following:

- *Design with and for older adults:* It is difficult or impossible to imagine and accurately design for experiences outside of our own. The involvement of older adults early and throughout the design process is crucial to avoid the creation of exergames that are not tailored to the physical and cognitive capabilities of the population they are targeting. Older adults have a range of different abilities that are not necessarily age or disease dependent, therefore making it difficult to capture generalizations or stereotypes. Involving older adults in the design process ensures that aspects such as motivators, preferences, and previous experiences (gaming and otherwise) can be incorporated into the design choices; therefore improving the sense of familiarity and interest when playing the games [74]. UCD processes (see Section 7.1) have been found to be effective in producing the targeted healthcare outcomes in serious games used for healthy lifestyle promotion [28].
- *Create personalized and adaptive experiences*: Tailoring gameplay to individual needs and preferences is one of the key aspects that will enable exergames to transition from an experimental interactive routine for physical activity promotion and rehabilitation toward a more widely and accepted technique to assist aging. Commercially available exergames (e.g., Wii, Kinect) have limited possibilities to be tailored to individual needs. The design of custom-made exergames, empowered with system intelligence (e.g., machine learning), allows the creation of adaptive experiences that can be beneficial to improving their effectiveness with older adults [115]. Therefore, adaptation modalities based on game performance [104], cardiovascular responses [72], or kinematic variables [101] should be implemented and integrated in novel exergaming systems to create truly personalized and tailored experiences (see Section 7.5).
- *Demonstrate effectiveness*: A large portion of studies published in the field of exergaming to support aging have been conducted in interventions lasting a few weeks (nine weeks on average). Researchers have been lengthening the duration of the interventions to better understand the long-term effects of exergaming, including studying how robust the intervention is (i.e., whether detected

improvements persist for a length of time after the exergame is taken away). More research has to be done to identify and remove biases, such as the novelty effect, as well as barriers such as usability issues (e.g., learning curve) to ascertain the true effects of exergames with older adults [121].

7.8 Key areas for future work

We believe there are two areas that are a priority for research in this field: (1) Getting systems in the hands of therapists and end-users and (2) Creating user-friendly tools for content creation and prototyping.

- *Getting systems in the hands of therapists and end-users:* Like many areas of cutting-edge research, while there is much excitement about the topic, few systems have transitioned out of the research lab into successfully adoption by the targeted population. With modern VR-based systems there is an advantage over wholly prototypical technology; VR-based interventions usually run on commercially available hardware; thus the main barriers to deployment are less than those of completely prototypical technology. Namely, the challenge lies in establishing efficacy and deploying the software in a way that is accessible for uptake by therapists and other end-users. To support this, more attention should be paid to designing gaming systems that have characteristics that will enable an easier move out of the research lab. Considering and supporting aspects such as accessible hardware, modifiable/scalable content, and integration to user-access platforms will help to facilitate technology uptake. Involving industry partners when possible is a good approach as they bring perspectives and expertise regarding real-world deployment, sustainable use, and related support.
- *Tools for content creation and prototyping:* True widespread and rapid development requires systematic adoption of flexible software and hardware tools that can be used to create content (e.g., virtual environments) and prototypes that can be tailored to the unique physical and cognitive abilities of older adults with relatively low effort. This will allow healthcare professionals with little-to-no technical background (e.g., physical therapists) to create prototypes that are more aligned with the real-world, which supports adoption and use. Previous research has shown how throughout the use of Do-It-Yourself (DIY) methodologies, exercise therapists can create/modify prototypes of digital and interactive technologies to support older adults [100]. Efforts such as these need to be expanded to enable more equitable engagement in the process by a disparate stakeholder.

7.9 Conclusions

Exergames to support aging is an exciting, promising, and rapidly expanding field that is engaging multidisciplinary teams from around the world. Their versatility and applications are only limited by our imaginations. This chapter provided a review of how serious games, and in particular exergames, can be a versatile and complementary tool in promoting better health and wellbeing for older adults. Key terminology and technological aspects were covered in this chapter, allowing better understanding of the multiple aspects that are commonly used as well as ways of creating exergames that are more likely to be adopted and used. The information in Appendix 1 and summarized in Table 7.1 constitutes an overview of validated tools that can be used to objectively assess the effects of serious games. The use of evaluation tools such as these and reporting findings in a complete, systematic way is key to providing greater evidence of the impact of serious games, which can then support better design as well as their uptake and use.

The future of the field is exciting and promising, especially with new healthcare challenges appearing (e.g., physical distancing, remote access) and the possibility of specialized games to be more sophisticated, better connected, and more effective in eliciting the desired responses and producing the expected benefits. Exploring the many opportunities for creating more personalized, effective, and fun games for this population will be an engaging area of research for many years to come.

John Edison Muñoz is a game designer and interface technologist specialized in the use of physiological signals to optimize the user experience while using interactive systems. John is currently a postdoctoral fellow at the University of Waterloo carrying out research in the fields of assistive technology, human-robot interaction, and virtual reality. John as codesigned multiple games that can be used in healthcare scenarios such as exercise promotion in older adults, self-regulation training in children with special needs, and cognitive training in neurorehabilitation.

Maria Fernanda Montoya is an engineer specialized in human computer interaction applications for rehabilitation and sports. She recently finished her master's in electrical engineering, developing physiological adaptive systems for upper arms rehabilitation. Maria's current research interest involves the use of the virtual reality environments in motor rehabilitation, the design and development of games and virtual scenarios targeting older adults with and without motor impairments.

Jennifer Boger is passionate about creating new ways to provide more inclusive, equitable support for health, wellbeing, and quality of life for older adults. Her team at the Intelligent Technologies for Wellness and Independent Living lab (www.itwil.ca) engages in transdisciplinary collaboration and user-driven design practices that blend state-of-the art knowledge from computer science, engineering, and rehabilitation sciences to create internationally renowned intelligent assistive technologies to support graceful aging. Over the past 15 years Jennifer has been a researcher on 38 projects and is an author of over 100 peer-reviewed publications.

References

[1] C. Abras, D. Maloney-Krichmar, J. Preece, et al., User-centered design, in: W. Bainbridge (Ed.), Encyclopedia of Human-Computer Interaction, 37, Sage Publications, Thousand Oaks, 2004, pp. 445–456.

[2] M. Adcock, F. Sonder, A. Schattin, F. Gennaro, E.D. de Bruin, A usability study of a multicomponent video game-based training for older adults, Eur. Rev. Aging Phys. Activ. 17 (1) (2020) 3.

[3] A. Al Mahmud, O. Mubin, S. Shahid, J.B. Martens, Designing social games for children and older adults: two related case studies, Entertain. Comput. 1 (3-4) (2010) 147–156.

[4] C. Anderson-Hanley, P.J. Arciero, A.M. Brickman, J.P. Nimon, N. Okuma, S.C. Westen, M.E. Merz, B.D. Pence, J.A. Woods, A.F. Kramer, et al., Exergaming and older adult cognition: a cluster randomized clinical trial, Am. J. Prev. Med. 42 (2) (2012) 109–119.

[5] J.A. Anguera, J. Boccanfuso, J.L. Rintoul, O. Al-Hashimi, F. Faraji, J. Janowich, E. Kong, Y. Larraburo, C. Rolle, E. Johnston, et al., Video game training enhances cognitive control in older adults, Nature 501 (7465) (2013) 97–101.

[6] P. Arias, V. Robles-Garc a, G. Sanmart n, J. Flores, J. Cudeiro, Virtual reality as a tool for evaluation of repetitive rhythmic movements in the elderly and Parkinson's disease patients, PloS One 7 (1) (2012) e30021.

[7] A.A.B. Arntzen, Game based learning to enhance cognitive and physical capabilities of elderly people: concepts and requirements, Int. J. Inf. Commun. Eng. 5 (12) (2011) 1778–1782.

[8] J.M.R. Bacha, G.C.V. Gomes, T.B. de Freitas, L.A.P. Viveiro, K.G. da Silva, G.C. Bueno, E.M. Varise, C. Torriani-Pasin, A.C. Alonso, N.M.S. Luna, et al., Effects of kinect adventures games versus conventional physical therapy on postural control in elderly people: a randomized controlled trial, Games Health J. 7 (1) (2018) 24–36.

[9] S. Ballesteros, A. Prieto, J. Mayas, P. Toril, C. Pita, L. Ponce de Leon, J.M. Reales, J. Waterworth, Brain training with non-action video games enhances aspects of cognition in older adults: a randomized controlled trial, Front. Aging Neurosci. 6 (2014) 277.

[10] C. Basak, W.R. Boot, M.W. Voss, A.F. Kramer, Can training in a real-time strategy video game attenuate cognitive decline in older adults?, Psychol. Aging 23 (4) (2008) 765.

[11] D. Bavelier, C.S. Green, A. Pouget, P. Schrater, Brain plasticity through the life span: learning to learn and action video games, Annu. Rev. Neurosci. 35 (2012) 391–416.

[12] J. Boger, P. Jackson, M. Mulvenna, J. Sixsmith, A. Sixsmith, A. Mihailidis, P. Kontos, J. Miller Polgar, A. Grigorovich, S. Martin, Principles for fostering the transdisciplinary development of assistive technologies, Disabil. Rehabil. Assist. Technol. 12 (5) (2017) 480–490.

[13] C. Boletsis, S. McCallum, Augmented reality cubes for cognitive gaming: preliminary usability and game experience testing, Int. J. Serious Games 3 (1) (2016) 3–18.

[14] E. Brox, S.T. Konstantinidis, G. Evertsen, User-centered design of serious games for older adults following 3 years of experience with exergames for seniors: a study design, JMIR Serious Games 5 (1) (2017) e2.

[15] E. Brox, L.F. Luque, G.J. Evertsen, J.E.G. Hernandez, Exergames for elderly: Social exergames to persuade seniors to increase physical activity, In: Proc. 5th International Conference on Pervasive Computing Technologies for Healthcare (PervasiveHealth) and Workshops, IEEE, 2011, pp. 546–549.

[16] B., Bushman, of Sports Medicine, A.C., ACSM's Complete Guide to Fitness & Health, 2E, Human Kinetics (2017).

[17] M. Cacciata, A. Stromberg, J.A. Lee, D. Sorkin, D. Lombardo, S. Clancy, A. Nyamathi, L.S. Evangelista, Effect of exergaming on health-related quality of life in older adults: a systematic review, Int. J. Nurs. Stud. 93 (2019) 30–40.
[18] S.T. Chen, Y.G.L. Huang, I.T. Chiang, Using somatosensory video games to promote quality of life for the elderly with disabilities, Proc. IEEE Fourth International Conference On Digital Game And Intelligent Toy Enhanced Learning, IEEE, 2012, pp. 258–262.
[19] A. Chesham, P. Wyss, R.M. Muri, U.P. Mosimann, T. Nef, What older people like to play: genre preferences and acceptance of casual games, JMIR Serious Games 5 (2) (2017) e8.
[20] A. Chirico, T. Giovannetti, P. Neroni, S. Simone, L. Gallo, F. Galli, F. Gian-camilli, M. Predazzi, F. Lucidi, G. De Pietro, et al., Virtual reality for the assessment of everyday cognitive functions in older adults: an evaluation of the virtual reality action test and two interaction devices in a 91-year-old woman, Front. Psychol. 11 (2020).
[21] K.H. Cho, K.J. Lee, C.H. Song, Virtual-reality balance training with a video-game system improves dynamic balance in chronic stroke patients, Tohoku J. Exp. Med. 228 (1) (2012) 69–74.
[22] F. Clay, D. Howett, J. FitzGerald, P. Fletcher, D. Chan, A. Price, Use of immersive virtual reality in the assessment and treatment of Alzheimer's disease: a systematic review, J. Alzheimer's Dis (2020) 1–21 Preprint.
[23] G. Corno, S. Bouchard, H. Forget, Usability assessment of the virtual multitasking test (V-MT) for elderly people, Annu. Rev. Cyberther. Telemed. 199 (2014) 168–172.
[24] R.Q.M. da Costa, J.E. Pompeu, D.D. de Mello, E. Moretto, F.Z. Rodrigues, M.D. Dos Santos, R. Nitrini, F. Morganti, S.M.D. Brucki, Two new virtual reality tasks for the assessment of spatial orientation preliminary results of tolerability, sense of presence and usability, Dementia Neuropsychol. 12 (2) (2018) 196.
[25] J.K. Dal Jae Im, Y.J. Kim, S. Cho, Y.K. Cho, T. Lim, H.S. Lee, H.J. Kim, Y.J. Kang, Utility of a three-dimensional interactive augmented reality program for balance and mobility rehabilitation in the elderly: a feasibility study, Ann. Rehabil. Med. 39 (3) (2015) 462.
[26] K. Daniel, Wii-HAB for pre-frail older adults, Rehabil. Nurs. 37 (4) (2012) 195–201.
[27] B.M. De Queiroz, A.F. Borgatto, A.R. Barbosa, A.V. Guimaraes, Exergame vs. aerobic exercise and functional fitness of older adults: a randomized controlled trial, J. Phys. Educ. Sport 17 (2) (2017) 740.
[28] A. DeSmet, D. Thompson, T. Baranowski, A. Palmeira, M. Verloigne, I. De Bourdeaudhuij, Is participatory design associated with the effectiveness of serious digital games for healthy lifestyle promotion? A meta-analysis, J. Med. Internet Res. 18 (4) (2016) e94.
[29] L. Desteghe, K. Kluts, J. Vijgen, P. Koopman, D. Dilling-Boer, J. Schurmans, P. Dendale, H. Heidbuchel, The health buddies app as a novel tool to improve adherence and knowledge in atrial fibrillation patients: a pilot study, JMIR MHealth UHealth 5 (7) (2017) e98.
[30] G. Epelde, E. Carrasco, S. Rajasekharan, J.M. Jimenez, K. Vivanco, I. Gomez-Fraga, X. Valencia, J. Florez, J. Abascal, Universal remote delivery of rehabilitation: validation with seniors' joint rehabilitation therapy, Cybern. Syst. 45 (2) (2014) 109–122.
[31] A.L. Faria, M.S. Pinho, S.B. i Badia, Capturing expert knowledge for the personalization of cognitive rehabilitation: study combining computational modeling and a participatory design strategy, JMIR Rehabil. Assist. Technol. 5 (2) (2018) e10714.
[32] H. Fordell, K. Bodin, G. Bucht, J. Malm, A virtual reality test battery for assessment and screening of spatial neglect, Acta Neurol. Scand. 123 (3) (2011) 167–174.
[33] K. Gerling, P. Dickinson, K. Hicks, L. Mason, A.L. Simeone, K. Spiel, Virtual reality games for people using wheelchairs, Proc. CHI Conference on Human Factors in Computing Systems, 2020 1–11.
[34] J. Gerlowska, U. Skrobas, K. Grabowska-Aleksandrowicz, A. Korchut, S. Szklener, D. Szczesniak-Stanczyk, D. Tzovaras, K. Rejdak, Assessment of perceived attractiveness,

usability, and societal impact of a multimodal robotic assistant for aging patients with memory impairments, Front. Neurol. 9 (2018) 392.

[35] G.C.V. Gomes, M. do Socorro Simoes, S.M. Lin, J.M.R. Bacha, L.A.P. Viveiro, E.M. Varise, N.C. Junior, B. Lange, W. Jacob Filho, J.E. Pompeu, Feasibility, safety, acceptability, and functional outcomes of playing Nintendo Wii fit Plus^{TM} for frail older adults: a randomized feasibility clinical trial, Maturitas 118 (2018) 20–28.

[36] A.R. Goncalves, J.E. Munoz, E.R. Gouveia, M. da Silva Cameirao, S.B. i Badia, Effects of prolonged multidimensional fitness training with exergames on the physical exertion levels of older adults, Vis. Comput. (2019) 1–12.

[37] A.R. Gonçalves, E.R. Gouveia, M.S. Cameirão, S.B.I Badia, "Automating senior fitness testing through gesture detection with depth sensors," IET International Conference on Technologies for Active and Assisted Living (TechAAL), 2015, pp. 1–6, doi: 10.1049/ic.2015.0132.

[38] G. Grossi, R. Lanzarotti, P. Napoletano, N. Noceti, F. Odone, Positive technology for elderly well-being: a review, Pattern Recognit. Lett. (2019).

[39] C.N. Harrington, J.Q. Hartley, T.L. Mitzner, W.A. Rogers, Assessing older adults' usability challenges using kinect-based exergames, Proc. International Conference on Human Aspects of IT for the Aged Population, Springer, 2015, pp. 488–499.

[40] J.P.O. Held, K. Yu, C. Pyles, J.M. Veerbeek, F. Bork, S.M. Heining, N. Navab, A.R. Luft, Augmented reality-based rehabilitation of gait impairments: case report, JMIR MHealth UHealth 8 (5) (2020) e17804.

[41] R.M. Himmelmeier, R. Nouchi, T. Saito, D. Burin, J. Wiltfang, R. Kawashima, Study protocol: does an acute intervention of high-intensity physical exercise followed by a brain training video game has immediate effects on brain activity of older people during stroop task in FMRI? A randomized controlled trial with crossover design, Front. Aging Neurosci. 11 (2019) 260.

[42] M. Hou, S. Banbury, C. Burns, Intelligent Adaptive Systems: An Interaction-Centered Design Perspective, CRC Press, Boca Raton, FL, 2014.

[43] Y. Hutzler, O. Korsensky, Y. Laufer, Rapid stepping test towards virtual visual objects: feasibility and convergent validity in older adults, Technol. Health Care 25 (1) (2017) 49–58.

[44] H. Huygelier, B. Schraepen, R. van Ee, V.V. Abeele, C.R. Gillebert, Acceptance of immersive head-mounted virtual reality in older adults, Sci. Rep. 9 (1) (2019) 1–12.

[45] H.T. Jung, H. Lee, K. Kim, B. Kim, S. Park, T. Ryu, Y. Kim, S.I. Lee, Estimating mini mental state examination scores using game-specific performance values: a preliminary study, Proc. 40th Annual International Conference of the IEEE Engineering in Medicine and Biology Society (EMBC), IEEE, 2018, pp. 1518–1521.

[46] D.L. Kappen, P. Mirza-Babaei, L.E. Nacke, Older adults' physical activity and exergames: a systematic review, Int. J. Hum-Comput. Int. 35 (2) (2019) 140–167.

[47] N. Katajapuu, M. Luimula, Y.L. Theng, T.P. Pham, J. Li, A. Pyae, K. Sato, Benefits of exergame exercise on physical functioning of elderly people, Proc. 8th IEEE International Conference on Cognitive Infocommunications (CogInfo-Com), IEEE, 2017, pp. 000085–000090.

[48] P.M. Kato, The role of the researcher in making serious games for health, in: S. Arnab, I. Dunwell, K. Debattista (Eds.), Serious Games for Healthcare: Applications and Implications, IGI Global, PA, 2013, pp. 213–231.

[49] B. Keshavarz, R. Ramkhalawansingh, B. Haycock, S. Shahab, J. Campos, Comparing simulator sickness in younger and older adults during simulated driving under different multisensory conditions, Transp. Res. F Traffic Psychol. Behav. 54 (2018) 47–62.

[50] R., Kizony, P., Weiss, M., Shahar, D., Rand: Theragame-A Home Based Virtual Reality Rehabilitation System. Esbjerg, Denmark (2006).

[51] D.K. Kumar, S.P. Arjunan, Human-Computer Interface Technologies for the Motor Impaired, 12, CRC Press, Boca Raton FL, 2015.

[52] K.E. Laver, B. Lange, S. George, J.E. Deutsch, G. Saposnik, M. Crotty, Virtual reality for stroke rehabilitation, Cochrane Database Syst. Rev. (11) (2017).

[53] D. Levac, S. Glegg, H. Colquhoun, P. Miller, F. Noubary, Virtual reality and active videogame-based practice, learning needs, and preferences: a cross-Canada survey of physical therapists and occupational therapists, Games Health J. 6 (4) (2017) 217–228.

[54] J. Li, M. Erdt, L. Chen, Y. Cao, S.Q. Lee, Y.L. Theng, The social effects of exergames on older adults: systematic review and metric analysis, J. Med. Internet Res. 20 (6) (2018) e10486.

[55] Li, S., Liu, S.: Functional Fitness for the Elderly. Ministry of Health and Welfare, Taipei (2008).

[56] Y. Li, J. Mu~noz, S. Mehrabi, L. Middleton, S. Cao, J. Boger, Multidisciplinary iterative design of exergames (MIDE): a framework for supporting the design, development, and evaluation of exergames for health, Proc. International Conference on Human-Computer Interaction, Springer, 2020, pp. 128–147.

[57] C.X. Lin, C. Lee, D. Lally, J.F. Coughlin, Impact of virtual reality (VR) experience on older adults' well-being, Proc. International Conference on Human Aspects of IT for the Aged Population, Springer, 2018, pp. 89–100.

[58] C.L. Liu, S.T. Uang, A study of sickness induced within a 3D virtual store and combated with fuzzy control in the elderly, Proc. 9th International Conference on Fuzzy Systems and Knowledge Discovery, IEEE, 2012, pp. 334–338.

[59] R. Llorens, J. Latorre, E. Noe, E.A. Keshner, Posturography using the Wii balance board™: a feasibility study with healthy adults and adults post-stroke, Gait Posture 43 (2016) 228–232.

[60] S. Macis, D. Loi, A. Ulgheri, D. Pani, G. Solinas, S. La Manna, V. Cestone, D. Guerri, L. Ra o, Design and usability assessment of a multi-device SOA-based telecare framework for the elderly, IEEE J. Biomed. Health Inform. 24 (1) (2019) 268–279.

[61] P. Maillot, A. Perrot, A. Hartley, Effects of interactive physical-activity video-game training on physical and cognitive function in older adults, Psychol. Aging 27 (3) (2012) 589.

[62] R.L. Mandryk, M.V. Birk, The potential of game-based digital biomarkers for modeling mental health, JMIR Ment. Health 6 (4) (2019) e13485.

[63] E.C. Marinelli, W.A. Rogers, Identifying potential usability challenges for Xbox 360 kinect exergames for older adults, Proc. Human Factors and Ergonomics Society Annual Meeting, Los Angeles, CA, 58, SAGE Publications Sage CA, 2014, pp. 1247–1251.

[64] S. McCallum, C. Boletsis, A taxonomy of serious games for dementia, in: B. Schouten, S. Fedtke, T. Bekker, M. Schijven, A. Gekker (Eds.), Games for Health, Springer, Cham, 2013, pp. 219–232.

[65] J.S. McGee, C. van der Zaag, J.G. Buckwalter, M. Thiebaux, A. Van Rooyen, U. Neumann, D. Sisemore, A.A. Rizzo, Issues for the assessment of visuospatial skills in older adults using virtual environment technology, CyberPsychol. Behav. 3 (3) (2000) 469–482.

[66] R. Mellecker, E.J. Lyons, T. Baranowski, Disentangling fun and enjoyment in exergames using an expanded design, play, experience framework: a narrative review, Games Health J. 2 (3) (2013) 142–149.

[67] A. Mirelman, I. Maidan, J.E. Deutsch, Virtual reality and motor imagery: promising tools for assessment and therapy in Parkinson's disease, Mov. Disord. 28 (11) (2013) 1597–1608.

[68] J. Mishra, A. Gazzaley, Closed-loop cognition: the next frontier arrives, Trends Cogn. Sci. 19 (5) (2015) 242–243.

[69] K.I. Molina, N.A. Ricci, S.A. de Moraes, M.R. Perracini, Virtual reality using games for improving physical functioning in older adults: a systematic review, J. Neuroeng. Rehabil. 11 (1) (2014) 156.

[70] A.G. Money, A. Atwal, E. Boyce, S. Gaber, S. Windeatt, K. Alexandrou, Falls sensei: a serious 3D exploration game to enable the detection of extrinsic home fall hazards for older adults, BMC Med. Inform. Decis. Mak. 19 (1) (2019) 85.

[71] F. Mueller, M.R. Gibbs, F. Vetere, Taxonomy of exertion games, Proc. Australasian Conference on Computer-Human Interaction: Designing for Habitus and Habitat, 2008 263–266.

[72] J.E. Muñoz, M. Cameir~ao, S. Bermudez i Badia, E.R. Gouveia, Closing the loop in exergaming-health benefits of biocybernetic adaptation in senior adults, Proc. Annual Symposium on Computer-Human Interaction in Play, 2018 329–339.

[73] J.E. Muñoz, S. Cao, J. Boger, Kinematically adaptive exergames: Personalizing exercise therapy through closed-loop systems, Proc. IEEE International Conference on Artificial Intelligence and Virtual Reality, 2019 118–125.

[74] J.E. Munoz, A. Goncalves, E. Rubio Gouveia, M.S. Cameirao, S. Bermudez i Badia, Lessons learned from gamifying functional fitness training through human-centered design methods in older adults, Games Health J. 8 (6) (2019) 387–406.

[75] Y. Nagano, K. Ishida, T. Tani, M. Kawasaki, M. Ikeuchi, Short and long-term effects of exergaming for the elderly, Springerplus 5 (1) (2016) 1–10.

[76] B.B. Neves, F. Vetere, Ageing and emerging digital technologies, in: B.B. Neves, F. Vetere (Eds.), Ageing and Digital Technology, Springer, Cham, 2019, pp. 1–14.

[77] T.N.T. Nguyen, S. Karwita, Y. Liangkun, S. Yongjie, Hacking occupational therapy tools for center-based care, Proc. ACM Conference Companion Publication on Designing Interactive Systems, 2018 111–115.

[78] S. Nikitina, D. Didino, M. Baez, F. Casati, Feasibility of virtual tablet-based group exercise among older adults in Siberia: findings from two pilot trials, JMIR MHealth UHealth 6 (2) (2018) e40.

[79] T. Okano, D. Kitakoshi, M. Suzuki, A preliminary study on preventive care system based on game playing with communication robots, Proc. Conference on Technologies and Applications of Artificial Intelligence, IEEE, 2013, pp. 84–89.

[80] F.R. Ortega, F. Abyarjoo, A. Barreto, N. Rishe, M. Adjouadi, Interaction Design for 3D User Interfaces: The World of Modern Input Devices for Research, Applications, and Game Development, CRC Press, Boca Raton, FL, 2016.

[81] E.C. Park, S.G. Kim, C.W. Lee, The effects of virtual reality game exercise on balance and gait of the elderly, J. Phys. Ther. Sci. 27 (4) (2015) 1157–1159.

[82] T. Park, I. Hwang, U. Lee, S.I. Lee, C. Yoo, Y. Lee, H. Jang, S.P. Choe, S. Park, J. Song, Exerlink: enabling pervasive social exergames with heterogeneous exercise devices, Proc. 10th International Conference on Mobile Systems, Applications, and Services, 2012 15–28.

[83] T.D. Parsons, A.A. Rizzo, Initial validation of a virtual environment for assessment of memory functioning: virtual reality cognitive performance assessment test, CyberPsychol. Behav. 11 (1) (2008) 17–25.

[84] E. Pedroli, L. Greci, D. Colombo, S. Serino, P. Cipresso, S. Arlati, M. Mondellini, L. Boilini, V. Giussani, K. Goulene, et al., Characteristics, usability, and users experience of a system combining cognitive and physical therapy in a virtual environment: positive bike, Sensors 18 (7) (2018) 2343.

[85] E. Pedroli, S. Serino, P. Cipresso, F. Pallavicini, I.A.C. Giglioli, E. Guasta erro, A. Gaggioli, G. Riva, Neglect app. usability of a new application for assessment and rehabilitation of neglect, Proc. 3rd 2015 Workshop on ICTs for Improving Patients Rehabilitation Research Techniques, 2015 139–143.

[86] W. Peng, J.H. Lin, J. Crouse, Is playing exergames really exercising? A meta-analysis of energy expenditure in active video games, Cyberpsychol. Behav. Soc. Netw. 14 (11) (2011) 681–688.

[87] G. Plancher, P. Piolino, Virtual reality for assessment of episodic memory in normal and pathological aging, in: R.L. Kane, T.D. Parsons (Eds.), The Role of Technology

in Clinical Neuropsychology, Oxford University Press, Oxford, 2017, pp. 237–260.
[88] A. Plechata, V. Sahula, D. Fayette, I. Fajnerova, Age-related differences with immersive and non-immersive virtual reality in memory assessment, Front. Psychol. 10 (2019) 1330.
[89] R. Pro tt, B. Lange, C. Chen, C. Winstein, A comparison of older adults' subjective experiences with virtual and real environments during dynamic balance activities, J. Aging Phys. Activ. 23 (1) (2015) 24–33.
[90] A. Pyae, T.N. Liukkonen, T. Saarenpaa, M. Luimula, P. Granholm, J. Smed, When Japanese elderly people play a Finnish physical exercise game: a usability study, J. Usability Stud. 11 (4) (2016) 131–152.
[91] P.A. Rego, P.M. Moreira, L.P. Reis, Proposal of an extended taxonomy of serious games for health rehabilitation, Games Health J. 7 (5) (2018) 302–309.
[92] G. Riva, A. Gaggioli, D. Villani, A. Preziosa, F. Morganti, R. Corsi, G. Faletti, L. Vezzadini, Neurovr: an open source virtual reality platform for clinical psychology and behavioral neurosciences, Stud. Health Technol. Inform. 125 (2007) 394–399.
[93] D. Rosenberg, C.A. Depp, I.V. Vahia, J. Reichstadt, B.W. Palmer, J. Kerr, G. Norman, D.V. Jeste, Exergames for subsyndromal depression in older adults: a pilot study of a novel intervention, Am. J. Geriatr. Psychiatry 18 (3) (2010) 221–226.
[94] B. Sawyer, P. Smith, Serious games taxonomy, Slides from the Serious Games Summit at the Game Developers Conference, 5, 2008.
[95] A. Schwarz, C.M. Kanzler, O. Lambercy, A.R. Luft, J.M. Veerbeek, Systematic review on kinematic assessments of upper limb movements after stroke, Stroke 50 (3) (2019) 718–727.
[96] F.R. Sheu, Y.L. Lee, H.T. Hsu, N.S. Chen, Effects of gesture-based fitness games on functional fitness of the elders, Proc. IEEE 15th International Conference on Advanced Learning Technologies, IEEE, 2015, pp. 158–160.
[97] T.E. Shubert, J. Basnett, A. Chokshi, M. Barrett, R. Komatireddy, Are virtual rehabilitation technologies feasible models to scale an evidence-based fall prevention program? A pilot study using the kinect camera, JMIR Rehabil. Assist. Technol. 2 (2) (2015) e10.
[98] J.M. Silva, A. El Saddik, An adaptive game-based exercising framework, Proc. IEEE International Conference on Virtual Environments, Human-Computer Interfaces and Measurement Systems Proceedings, IEEE, 2011, pp. 1–6.
[99] M. Slater, M.V. Sanchez-Vives, Enhancing our lives with immersive virtual reality, Front. Robot. AI 3 (2016) 74.
[100] K. Slegers, K. Kouwenberg, T. Loucova, R. Daniels, Makers in healthcare: The role of occupational therapists in the design of DIY assistive technology, Proc. CHI Conference on Human Factors in Computing Systems, 2020 1–11.
[101] J.D. Smeddinck, S. Siegel, M. Herrlich, Adaptive difficulty in exergames for Parkinson's disease patients, Proc. Graphics Interface, Regina, Saskatchewan, Canada, 2013 141–148.
[102] A.V. Soares, N.B. Junior, M. Hounsell, E. Marcelino, G.M. Rossito, Y.S. Junior, A serious game developed for physical rehabilitation of frail elderly. European research in telemedicine/La Recherche Europeenne en, Telemedecine 5 (2) (2016) 45–53.
[103] A. Sonderegger, S. Schmutz, J. Sauer, The influence of age in usability testing, Appl. Ergon. 52 (2016) 291–300.
[104] A. Streicher, J.D. Smeddinck, Personalized and adaptive serious games, in: R. Dörner, S. Göbel, M. Kickmeier Rust, M. Masuch, K. Zweig (Eds.), Entertainment Computing and Serious Games, Springer, Cham, 2016, pp. 332–377.
[105] E.A. Suma, B. Lange, A.S. Rizzo, D.M. Krum, M. Bolas, Faast: The Flexible action and articulated skeleton toolkit, Proc. IEEE Virtual Reality Conference, IEEE, 2011, pp. 247–248.

[106] L. Taylor, N. Kerse, J. Klenk, R. Borotkanics, R. Maddison, Exergames to improve the mobility of long-term care residents: a cluster randomized controlled trial, Games Health J. 7 (1) (2018) 37–42.
[107] L.M. Taylor, R. Maddison, L.A. Pfae i, J.C. Rawstorn, N. Gant, N.M. Kerse, Activity and energy expenditure in older people playing active video games, Arch. Phys. Med. Rehabil. 93 (12) (2012) 2281–2286.
[108] J. Tromp, M. Akbal, L. Pohl, S. Krohn, E.M. Quinque, F. Klotzsche, A. Vill-ringer, M. Gaebler, Openvirtualobjects: an open set of standardized and validated 3d household objects for virtual reality-based research, diagnostics, and therapy, Proc. International Conference on Virtual Rehabilitation (ICVR), IEEE, 2019, pp. 1–2.
[109] P.T. Trzepacz, H. Hochstetler, S. Wang, B. Walker, A.J. Saykin, A.D.N. Initiative, et al., Relationship between the Montreal cognitive assessment and mini-mental state examination for assessment of mild cognitive impairment in older adults, BMC Geriatr. 15 (1) (2015) 107.
[110] T.H. Tsai, K.C. Tseng, A.M. Wong, H.J. Chang, A study exploring the usability of an exergaming platform for senior fitness testing, Health Inform. J. 26 (2) (2020) 963–980.
[111] S. Tu, S. Wong, J.R. Hodges, M. Irish, O. Piguet, M. Hornberger, Lost in spatial translation. A novel tool to objectively assess spatial disorientation in Alzheimer's disease and frontotemporal dementia, Cortex 67 (2015) 83–94.
[112] C. Tuena, E. Pedroli, P.D. Trimarchi, A. Gallucci, M. Chiappini, K. Goulene, A. Gaggioli, G. Riva, F. Lattanzio, F. Giunco, et al., Usability issues of clinical and research applications of virtual reality in older people: a systematic review, Front. Hum. Neurosci. 14 (2020) 93.
[113] Z. Saenz-de Urturi, B. Garc a Zapirain, A. Mendez Zorrilla, Elderly user experience to improve a kinect-based game playability, Behav. Inf. Technol. 34 (11) (2015) 1040–1051.
[114] T. Vanbellingen, S.J. Filius, T. Ny eler, E.E. van Wegen, Usability of videogame-based dexterity training in the early rehabilitation phase of stroke patients: a pilot study, Front. Neurol. 8 (2017) 654.
[115] A. Velazquez, A.I. Mart nez-Garc a, J. Favela, S.F. Ochoa, Adaptive exergames to support active aging: an action research study, Pervasive Mob. Comput. 34 (2017) 60–78.
[116] A. Vourvopoulos, A.L. Faria, M.S. Cameirao, S.B. i Badia, Rehabnet: a distributed architecture for motor and cognitive neuro-rehabilitation, Proc. IEEE 15th International Conference on e-Health Networking, Applications and Services (Healthcom 2013), IEEE, 2013, pp. 454–459.
[117] S.P. Walz, S. Deterding, The Gameful World: Approaches, Issues, Applications, MIT Press, Cambridge, MA, 2015.
[118] V. Wattanasoontorn, I. Boada, R. Garc a, M. Sbert, Serious games for health, Entertain. Comput. 4 (4) (2013) 231–247.
[119] D. Webster, O. Celik, Systematic review of kinect applications in elderly care and stroke rehabilitation, J. Neuroeng. Rehabil. 11 (1) (2014) 108.
[120] G. Dermody, L. Whitehead, G. Wilson, C. Glass, The role of virtual reality in improving health outcomes for community-dwelling older adults: systematic review, J. Med. Internet Res. 22 (6) (2020) e17331.
[121] W. Xu, H.N. Liang, N. Baghaei, B. Wu Berberich, Y. Yue, Health benefits of digital videogames for the aging population: a systematic review, Games Health J. 9 (6) (2020) 389–404.
[122] A.S. Lu, H. Kharrazi, A state-of-the-art systematic content analysis of games for health, Games Health J. 7 (1) (2018) 1–15.
[123] A. DeSmet, D. Van Ryckeghem, S. Compernolle, T. Baranowski, D. Thompson, G. Crombez, I. De Bourdeaudhuij, A meta-analysis of serious digital games for healthy lifestyle promotion, Prev. Med. 69 (2014) 95–107.

[124] G. Mura, M.G. Carta, F. Sancassiani, S. Machado, L. Prosperini, Active exergames to improve cognitive functioning in neurological disabilities: a systematic review and meta-analysis, Eur. J. Phys. Rehab. Med. 54 (3) (2017) 450–462.

[125] T.B.F. Pacheco, C.S.P. de Medeiros, V.H.B. de Oliveira, E.R. Vieira, F.A.C de Cavalcanti, Effectiveness of exergames for improving mobility and balance in older adults: a systematic review and meta-analysis, Syst. Rev. 9 (1) (2020) 1–14.

[126] Q. Fang, P. Ghanouni, S.E. Anderson, H. Touchett, R. Shirley, F. Fang, C. Fang, Effects of exergaming on balance of healthy older adults: a systematic review and meta-analysis of randomized controlled trials, Games Health J. 9 (1) (2020) 11–23.

[127] D. Kaufman, M. Ma, L. Sauve, L. Renaud, E. Duplaa, Benefits of digital gameplay for older adults: does game type make a difference?, Int. J. Aging Res. 2 (4) (2019).

[128] M.T. Schultheis, R.R. Mourant, Virtual reality and driving: the road to better assessment for cognitively impaired populations, Presence Teleoperators Virtual Environ 10 (4) (2001) 431–439, doi:https://doi.org/10.1162/1054746011470271.

CHAPTER

8

Big Data, Big Data Analytics application to Smart home technologies and services for geriatric rehabilitation

Matthew Willetts, Anthony S. Atkins, Clare Stanier

School of Digital, Technologies and Art, Staffordshire University, Stoke-on-Trent, United Kingdom

LEARNING OBJECTIVES

- What are the challenges associated with an elderly population and associated rising healthcare costs and the application of Ambient Assisted Living (AAL) using sensor technology in Smart homes to support geriatric rehabilitation?
- What is meant by Big Data and to be able to distinguish the different categories of Big Data such as machine-generated data; human-generated data and business-generated data and its continued dramatic increase, particularly in IoT sensor technology and its application to geriatric rehabilitation.
- What is Big Data Analytics and how it differs from traditional Business Intelligence solutions using sensor technology in geriatric rehabilitation.
- A proposed monitoring solution using Big Data Analytics in a Smart home for geriatric rehabilitation by retrofitting existing homes with sensor technology.

8.1 Introduction

A major global challenge resulting from an increasingly elderly population is rising healthcare costs. Smart homes could provide a cost-effective, nonobtrusive solution allowing elderly and disabled residents to remain

Smart Home Technologies and Services for Geriatric Rehabilitation
DOI: https://doi.org/10.1016/B978-0-32-385173-2.00001-1

in their homes for longer [1]. Smart homes are houses with always on connections that generate immense volumes of valuable data from a variety of Smart devices and appliances connected to an Internet of Things (IoT) system [2]. Ambient-assisted living (AAL) environments are an integration of stand-alone assistive technologies, solutions, and services, and Smart homes are classified as IoT technology for the AAL domain [3]. The technologies utilized within a Smart home include: environmental sensors to capture parameters applicable to the homes and its residents relating to elements such as light, temperature, air quality, weather conditions, pressure, and movement; personal sensors including wearable technology; controllers and gateways; actuators and Smart appliances; and software [1]. The Smart home approach could also assist with geriatric rehabilitation, which is described as: "*a multidisciplinary set of evaluative, diagnostic, and therapeutic interventions whose purpose is to restore functional ability or enhance residual functional capability in elderly people with disabling impairments*" [4, p.1].

The World Health Organization (WHO) [110] states that between 2015 and 2050 the proportion of the world's population over 60 years of age will almost double from 12% to 22%. The WHO [110, p. 1] also states: "*there is, however, little evidence to suggest that older people today are experiencing their later years in better health than their parents. While rates of severe disability have declined in high-income countries over the past 30 years, there has been no significant change in mild to moderate disability over the same period.*" The Office for National Statistics UK [5] reported that the UK population was projected to exceed 70 million by 2031 and reach 72.4 million by mid-2043. Over the next 25 years, the number of older people will increase, with the proportion of individuals aged 85 years and over projected to almost double [5]. An aging population has important consequences both economically and socially, as it requires more care, an increase in the number of qualified people to support them, and the efficient management of health resources [6].

The data generated from Smart homes can be classified as Big Data, as these data have the characteristics of volume, velocity, and variety. For this reason sophisticated Big Data Analytics tools are required to unlock the potential of this dataset [2]. A data stream is defined as: "*a countably infinite sequence of elements and is used to represent data elements that are made available over time*" [7, p. 1], for example reading from the variety of sensors available in Smart homes. Yassine et al. [2] highlight that data streams from Smart homes present challenges for data processing and mining, as these Big Data sources change over time due to the changing behavior of the Smart home occupants; therefore scalable tools are required to process and analyze these data. Marjani et al. [8] state that different types of analytics are used depending on the requirements of IoT applications, for example real-time analytics are typically performed on sensor data as situations can change frequently, requiring rapid data analytics, whereas offline analytics can be utilized when a quick response is not required.

This chapter outlines what is meant by Big Data, explaining the types of Big Data, how Big Data has been adopted by companies and utilized to improve elderly care. The chapter also discusses Business Intelligence and Big Data Analytics to highlight the difference between these two types of analytic technologies, with examples provided of how Big Data Analytics has achieved measurable benefits for companies that have adopted it.

8.2 AAL and Smart homes

The term Smart health refers to the utilization of conventional mobile devices such as mobile phones with wearable medical devices (including blood pressure monitors, glucometers, smartwatches, and Smart contact lenses) and IoT gadgets (e.g., implantable or ingestible sensors) to facilitate continuous patient monitoring and treatment even when patients are at home [9]. Zeadally et al. [9, p. 2] state that: "*Smart health is expected to keep hospitalization expenses low and provide timely treatment for various medical conditions by placing IoT sensors on health monitoring equipment.*" This would suggest that Smart health can play a key role in addressing the challenges of an aging population.

AAL "*relates to intelligent systems of assistance for a better, healthier and safer life in the preferred living environment and covers concepts, products and services that interlink and improve new technologies and the social environment, with the aim of enhancing the quality of life for all elderly people in all stages of their life*" [10, p. vii]. Alsulami et al. [11] state that considerable research has clarified the needs and purpose of utilizing AAL technologies to monitor elderly people which include: the presence detection, sleep monitoring, fall detection, physiological parameter tracking (heart and breathing rates and gait), physical cleanliness, routine action monitoring (activity of daily living), Parkinson's disease, diabetes, Alzheimer's disease, posture detection, location tracking, health status, overweighing, medical guidance, treatment prescription, and economic reasons. AAL technologies include Smart homes, assistive robotics, mobile devices, e-textile, and wearable sensors [12]. Fig. 8.1 provides examples of proactive and integrated Smart home and AAL sensors that can provide exception alerts. For example, if a fall occurs, the care provider or next of kin can be notified via an SMS message or email.

Vadillo et al. [6, p. 348] define the Smart home concept in healthcare as: "*the integration of digital home technologies (devices, systems, and communications) with the necessary intelligence to recognize the health status and improve the person's quality of life (efficiently detecting and resolving situations dangerous to the person due to their health condition or their environment, or providing telemedicine services) and taking into account the needs and*

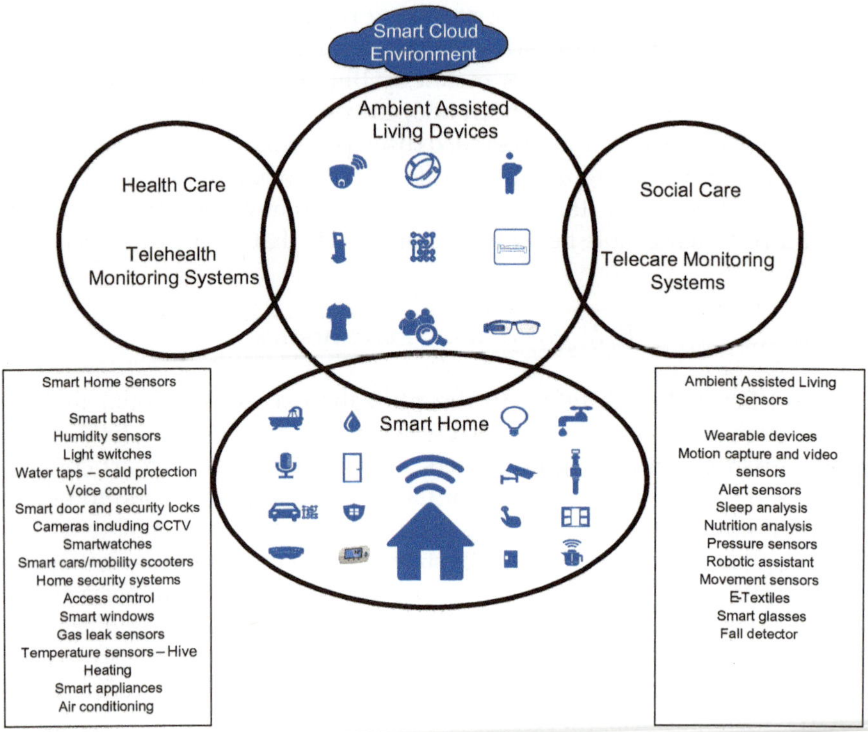

FIG. 8.1 Examples of Smart home and AAL devices.

expectations of its inhabitants." Technologies within Smart homes include: sensors to detect environmental factors including light, temperature, and motion; monitors; interfaces; appliances (such as heating and hot water systems), and other devices that are networked together, enabling the environment to be controlled on an automated or manual basis, locally or remotely [13]. AAL sensors include magnetic switches, temperature sensors, photosensors, pressure pad sensors, water flow sensors, infrared motion sensors, force sensors, smoke sensors, and biosensors [14]. From a healthcare perspective, Smart homes are a key enabler in improving the lives of residents. Alsulami and Atkins [12, p. 2] state that: "*the main benefits of Smart homes are improving comfort, performing medical rehabilitation, supervising mobility and physiological parameters, providing therapy, delivering convenience, improving security, and saving energy.*"

Choi, Choi, and Shon [15] suggest that the aim of AAL in residential spaces is to provide unobtrusive healthcare services by collecting information without conscious effort on the part of users and using this information to enable frequent monitoring that can support users in adjusting their behavior. The factors influencing adopting AAL technologies and the use of Smart watches to monitor heart rates in elderly people have been discussed previously by Alsulami and Atkins [12, 16], Alsulami et al. [17], and Alsulami et al. [11].

However, data privacy concerns may provide a challenge in the adoption of AAL technology. Uddin, Khaksar, and Torresen [14, p. 6] state that: *"the rights and legitimate concerns of the elderly must be balanced with the requirements of efficiently functioning healthcare systems. Thus, it is very important to determine the legal obligations that may arise from privacy and personal data collection issues. The data being captured from AAL sensors can be used to personally identify individuals, their activity, and their movements, therefore it is essential to obtain permission to capture this data and ensure it is stored securely."*

Age UK [18] states that the majority older people would prefer to live independently at home but the difficulty is that many of them live in substandard housing that requires adaptions, with one in five of all UK homes failing the decent homes test. They also estimate that the cost to the UK's National Health Service (NHS) of poor housing is £1.4 billion per year but £29,270 per person per year can be saved if a home can be modified to prevent the occupants moving to residential care. Therefore, one challenge associated with increasing the number of Smart homes to support geriatric rehabilitation is retrofitting the required sensors into existing homes. However, support is available in the United Kingdom from local authorities in the form of a needs assessment, which may result in recommendations including: home adaptations, assistive technology, or practical support at home (e.g., assistance with food shopping or medication prompts) [19]. Additionally, the types of housing stock vary between different countries. For example, it has been stated that the United Kingdom has the oldest housing stock in Europe and potentially the world, due to legacy homes built during the industrial revolution [20]. Another challenge are the differing building regulations, construction standards, and building materials that vary between countries, for example Meijer, Visscher, and Sheridan [21] compare building regulations between eight European countries. Between 2010 and 2019, 1.4 million new homes were registered to be built across the United Kingdom [22] compared with a total of 24.4 million dwellings in England [23]. This suggests that the majority of homes in the United Kingdom will require sensors to be retrofitted. Table 8.1 compares existing UK homes [20] and new house registrations [24] by type from 2017.

Table 8.2 shows a breakdown of UK properties by the period they were built [20], clearly showing that 54.76% of homes were built before 1964, suggesting that modernization work may be required in the majority of homes to facilitate Smart appliances. In comparison, 65.5% of Canada's homes were built from 1978 [25], as shown in Table 8.3 and consequently the buildings and home facilities are more modern.

Rafferty et al. [26] state that Smart homes require a large number of sensors to perform efficiently. This suggests that widespread adoption of

TABLE 8.1 A comparison between existing UK homes [20] and new UK house registrations [24] in 2017—modified by authors.

	Detached houses	Apartments	Semi-detached houses	Terraced houses	Bungalows	Total
2017 House Registrations (National House Building Council [24])	48,767	41,336	41,573	25,889	2,672	160,237
2017 UK Housing Stock [20]	5,107,000	5,958,000	7,129,000	7,829,000	2,512,000	28,535,000
Percentage of New builds to existing homes for 2017	0.95	0.69	0.58	0.33	0.11	0.56

the Smart home approach would be challenging because of scalability issues in retrofitting large numbers of sensors in addition to the financial cost of both installation and maintenance. Another major issue to consider is the longevity of devices with reports of security certificates expiring which may prevent devices from functioning [27]. Advances in network technology including 5G and Wi-Fi 6 can facilitate bigger and faster data streams in Smart homes [28]; however this also highlights that IoT devices have a limited lifespan and may need to be replaced as they become obsolete. 5G is an evolving technology which, once it becomes less dependent on 4G infrastructure, has been estimated to be up to 1000 times faster than 4G, with the potential to reach speeds between 10 and 50 Gbps which

TABLE 8.2 A comparison of UK dwellings by age (thousands of dwellings) for 2017 using data from Piddington et al. [20].

Dwelling age	United Kingdom	Percentage
Pre 1919	5,871	20.57
1919–1944	4,284	15.01
1945–1964	5,472	19.18
1965–1980	5,698	19.97
1981–1990	2,287	8.01
1990–2017	4,923	17.25
Total	28,536	100.00

TABLE 8.3 A comparison of Canadian homes by age (thousands of homes) for 2017 using data from Natural Resources Canada [25].

Age of homes	Canada	Percentage
Before 1946	1,594	10.25
1946–1960	1,164	7.49
1961–1977	2,599	16.72
1978–1983	1,544	9.93
1984–1995	3,098	19.93
1996–2000	1,047	6.73
2001–2005	1,294	8.33
2006–2010	1,318	8.48
2011–2015	1,196	7.69
2016–2017	691	4.45
Total	15,545	100.00

is fast enough to download an HD film in less than a second [29]. Average 5G speeds are around 130–240 Mbps, higher than the average home fiber broadband which are often less than 100 Mbps, therefore 5G broadband is now commercially available [29]. 5G offers the potential to resolve some of the scalability problems with Smart homes.

The increasing number of wearable sensors or sensors installed into Smart homes to support geriatric rehabilitation capture data including movement, biometrics, and the environment (temperature and humidity). These data are being generated at a high velocity, in a variety of formats resulting in an increasing magnitude of data to store. If multiple homes are being monitored by a third-party healthcare provider, this will present a challenge as these data will need to be stored by the provider into a storage solution that is scalable to support the huge volume of data. As the healthcare provider will need to be able to analyze the wellbeing of the residents and to identify when an anomaly occurs such as a fall or a heart attack, Big Data Analytics will be required to analyze the Big Data captured through the sensors.

8.3 Big Data

The term Big Data was initially used to describe data that are too large to be stored, processed, and analyzed using traditional business intelligence methods. Big Data is commonly associated with terabytes and petabytes of data [30], rather than gigabytes and smaller quantities. The International

Data Corporation (IDC) describes the Datasphere as the amount of data created, captured, and replicated in a specific year [31] and forecasts that the datasphere will increase from 33 zettabytes in 2018 to 175 zettabytes in 2025 [32]. The large quantities of data generated on a daily basis can partly be attributed to the growing number of Smart devices and social media, each producing data per individual transaction made [33].

Gartner uses the term "hype cycle" to describe the five phases new technologies progress through from initial conception to mainstream adoption: Innovation Trigger, Peak of Inflated Expectations, Trough of Disillusionment, Slope of Enlightenment, and Plateau of Productivity [34]. Big Data provides adopters with access to new sources of data and therefore led to high expectations in the years since its conception. Pence [35] states that one of the reasons that may explain these high expectations is that analysis of these data will allow more accurate identification of customer characteristics. It may be that Big Data has now moved from "hype" into a delivery phase as the adoption has moved to a plateau of productivity.

Big Data is defined as having a number of characteristics. Russom [36] stated that most definitions of Big Data focused on the volumes of data. However, there are other important characteristics and Russom [36] argues that the three characteristics (V's) that define Big Data are volume, velocity, and variety. The term "Big Data" has evolved beyond describing the "volume, variety, and velocity" of data and is now used to describe not only the data itself but the related technologies that capture, store, transform, and analyze the data to solve complex problems [37]. There is no agreed definition of Big Data [38] and the phrase has been described as a catch-all term for a wide selection of data [39]. Although later definitions have built on the Three V's, it is argued that they are only part of the full definition [40].

In the context of Big Data, volume refers to the magnitude of data, with data sizes frequently being quantified in terabytes and petabytes [41], with one terabyte being considered the minimum threshold of Big Data [42]. The volumes of Big Data could grow even larger to zettabytes, which is approximately equal to one thousand exabytes or one billion terabytes [43]. Velocity is the speed at which data are generated. Olszak and Mach-Król [44, p. 2] state that: "*in the contemporary global economy, the velocity dimension of big data is particularly important, as the speed at which an organization takes action is critical to its gaining a sustainable competitive advantage.*" Variety refers to the different sources and types of data, particularly structured and unstructured formats of data [45]. In the context of geriatric rehabilitation, the type of data most likely to be used for analysis is sensor data, for example tracking movements around the home. These data are likely to be generated in high volumes and at a high velocity and are typically unstructured.

Not all the authors agree that the Three V's accurately represent Big Data. Kitchin and McArdle [39] suggest that volume is a byproduct of velocity and the choice of dataset, referred to as exhaustivity; the example given is that sensor data may be produced at a high velocity, in real time, but the size of data produced may be very small. This has implications for the use of sensors in Smart homes although it should be noted that even if the data stream from a single Smart house is comparatively small, it is likely that the Smart home system would collect data from multiple homes or buildings in multiple occupation. The intention is that this proactive monitoring system would be a commercial operation under the auspices of a government agency and to be commercially viable it would need to be monitoring a substantial number of elderly homes in a specified region.

Additional V's have been added by organizations within the technology industry [46]. Table 8.4 summarizes some of the characteristics associated with Big Data.

Value was added by Oracle [42,51] arguing that data have no use until its value is discovered. The discovery process may involve analysts and other business users asking questions, finding patterns, making assumptions, and predicting behaviors. Other V's have been added including viability [47], visualization [48], and volatility [49]. The three V's have been extended with additional V's to produce four V's [50], five V's [47, 51], six V's [52], seven V's [48, 53], nine V's [54], and even ten V's [55]. Alsaig, Alagar, and Ormandjieva [56] identified 19 V's in their review of published work that describes various V's of Big Data. This has since been exceeded, satirically to 42 V's [57] and later to 51 [58] V's of Big Data, which has been suggested could reach 100 in the near future [58]. Fig. 8.2 displays examples of the combinations of the various V's over time. However, none of the additional V's appears to be used as consistently as the original three V's. Despite the popularity of adding additional V's and

TABLE 8.4 Kitchin's characteristics of Big Data [30, 39].

	Small data	Big Data
Volume	Limited to large	Very large—terabytes, petabytes or larger volumes of data
Velocity	Slow, freeze-framed/ bundled	Fast, continuous—data generated in real-time
Variety	Limited to wide—structured data	Wide—structured and unstructured data
Exhaustivity	Samples	Entire populations or systems
Resolution and indexicality	Course and weak to tight and strong	Tight and strong—highly detailed where possible
Relationality	Weak to strong	Strong—contain common fields that allow datasets to be joined
Extensionality and scalability	Low to middling	High—can add new fields easily and can expand in size rapidly

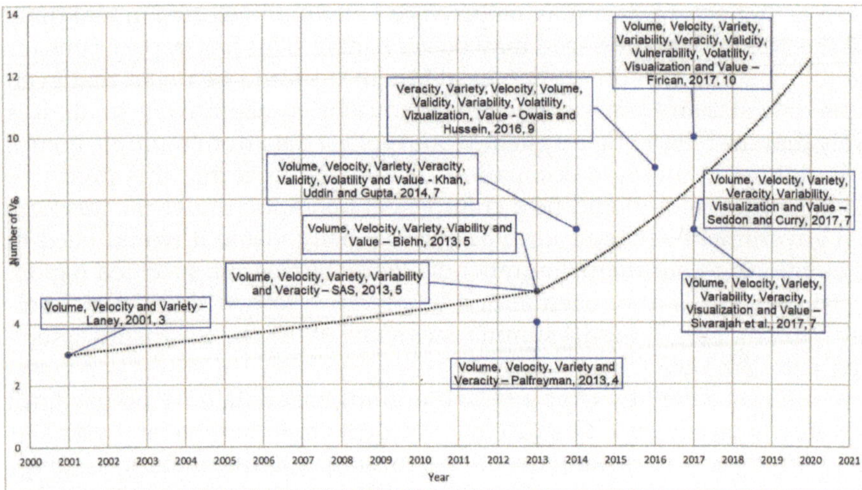

FIG. 8.2 Evolution of the V's of Big Data.

the changing combinations of V's, it could be argued that the three V's do not completely describe Big Data.

Pence [35] argues that complexity should be taken into account in addition to the three V's, giving the example of the increased use of personal genomes in the United States. Although the DNA of one individual would consume only 750 MB, to store the DNA of the entire USA population would require 222 petabytes. If the objective was to analyze the genome for one individual to find disease indicators, Big Data tools would be required due to the complexity of the interactions among the datasets. Complexity is also considered by other authors [45, 59–61], suggesting that this should be a key characteristic of Big Data. Complexity can then be considered as the fourth characteristic of Big Data, which already includes the three V's of volume, velocity, and variety.

Willetts, Atkins, and Stanier [46 p. 3034] define the term Big Data as: *"an umbrella term used to describe a wide range of technologies that capture, store, transform and analyze complex data sets which can be of a high volume, generated at a high velocity in a variety of formats."*

Big Data is generated from a wide range of sources. Saggi and Jain [62] define three categories of Big Data: machine-generated data that originate from sources including computer networks, sensors, satellites, audio, video, and streaming; human-generated data in the form of identification data and social media content; and business-generated data in the form of transactional, corporate and government agencies' data. IoT and Smart devices, including smartphones, are one of the prominent drivers for Big Data; each device typically contains digital sensors capable of capturing data, including cameras, audio recorders, compasses, gyroscopes, accelerometers, and GPS locators [38, 63]. Statista [64] reports that the number of smartphone users is expected to increase from 2.5 billion in 2016 to 3.8 billion in 2021, which will therefore further increase the volumes and speed of the data generated.

Dark data [65, 66] is the term used to describe underutilized datasets that exist both internally and externally within an organization. Internal dark data may include email archives, call center recordings, and documents. External dark data are the data found on social media sites including Facebook, YouTube, and Twitter, which may provide insight into customer's behaviors and views toward the company if utilized. The concept of dark data can be extended to describe activities that do not currently generate data in a usable form, for example the length of time taken to complete a daily activity. Questionnaires such as the Lawton Instrumental Activities of Daily Living Scale and the Katz Index of Independence in the Activities of Daily Living and the Timed up and Go Test are widely used elements in Geriatric Assessment [67]; the use of Smart home monitoring devices, with the user's consent, could provide valuable and possibly more accurate data.

Despite the perception that Big Data is expensive to adopt [48], there are options that do not require large upfront infrastructure costs. Big Data as a service (DaaS) is a cloud-based solution that bridges the storage and processing gap [68]. Many leading vendors offer DaaS solutions including Microsoft's Hadoop on Azure, Google Cloud Big Table, Amazon AWS with Elastic MapReduce, and Salesforce Analytics Cloud. These solutions provide the analytics, processing, storage, and visualization capabilities to transform data into insights.

Software tools are required to analyze the vast volumes of Big Data generated by Smart homes. Traditional data analytics are unable to process the huge volumes of Big Data, [69], therefore a range of Big Data Analytics solutions is required to analyze the unstructured data stored in a variety of sources including text and audio and video formats. Smart homes contain a diverse range of technology including wearable devices, temperature sensors, pressure sensors, and cameras which generate large volumes of structured and unstructured data that traditional Business Intelligence solutions do not have the capability to analyze. In addition to identifying how the Big Data generated by Smart homes will be stored, another challenge of Smart home implementation be adopting appropriate Big Data Analytics solutions to analyze the data.

8.4 Big Data Analytics

Big Data analytics is the process of extracting insights from Big Data using a variety of software tools and techniques, not achievable through traditional Business Intelligence solutions. Mikalef et al. [70] identified that several of the definitions of Big Data Analytics reviewed in their literature review focused on one of three categories: data and their defining characteristics; analytical procedures, tools, and techniques; and the business value of presentation of the data analysis. Mikalef et al. [71, p. 262] state that a widely used definition of Big Data Analytics is: "*a new generation of technologies and architectures, designed to economically extract value from very large volumes of a wide variety of data, by enabling high velocity capture, discovery and/or analysis.*" The wide variety of data referred to in this definition includes structured, semistructured, and unstructured data [46, 72].

Just as there is a lack of a universally accepted definition for Big Data and Big Data Analytics, there are different approaches to the classifications of Big Data Analytics [72]. Sivarajah et al. [48] describe the following five categories of Big Data Analytics:

- descriptive analytics
- inquisitive analytics
- predictive analytics
- prescriptive analytics
- pre-emptive analytics.

Descriptive analytics are the most common and well-understood category of analytics [73]. Descriptive analytics present the user with information about what has occurred historically and in a format that is easily interpreted including graphs, charts, maps, pie, and scatter diagrams, often in the style of a dashboard [74]. In the context of Smart Home data analytics, descriptive analytics would provide a record of the activities of the individual who is being monitored. Inquisitive analytics are used to probe data to understand why events are occurring [75]. This is achieved using techniques such as analytical drill down, statistical analysis, and factor analysis [48]. Inquisitive analytics could be used in a Smart home to examine, for example, factors that might be associated with falls. Predictive analytics refer to the techniques that use historical and current data to predict future outcomes and can be applied to all disciplines, for example it could be utilized to predict a customers' activity based on their purchase history and their social media activity [41]. Applying this to a Smart home, it might be possible to predict occupant behaviors and the consequences of behaviors. Sivarajah et al. [76, p. 276] state that prescriptive analytics: "*are performed to determine the cause-effect relationship among analytic results and business process optimization policies. Thus, for prescriptive analytics, organizations optimize their business process models based on the feedback provided by predictive analytic models.*" The technology is less mature than descriptive analytics but it is considered the next advance toward optimizing decision making for business performance improvement [77]. Kuttappa [78] provides examples of how prescriptive analytics have been successfully adopted in the healthcare industry, improving the quality of care by reducing wait times, reducing costs, and increasing transparency across functional areas. The final category of pre-emptive analytics is defined as: *"having the capacity to take precautionary actions on events that may undesirably influence the organizational performance, for example, identifying the possible perils and recommending mitigating strategies far ahead in time"* [48 p. 266]. Pre-emptive analytics is a developing area [48], for preemptive healthcare whereby intervention is taken at the earliest opportunity to prevent the patient's condition from deteriorating. An example of a monitoring system for wellbeing and e-Social care to support elderly residents in a healthcare environment is shown in Fig. 8.3. This type of e-Healthcare system provides an opportunity to reduce costs by supporting elderly people living at home. The system would assist in medication dispensing, changes in daily living patterns including the frequency of leaving the house, anomalies in daily activities such as sleeping, depression, memory loss, and toiletry habits. The system is agile and would allow the system to be customized, as illustrated in Fig. 8.3, for adding optional sensors and devices depending on the elderly residents' requirements and to future proof the system using a "plug and play" building system. To support this in the context of Smart homes, Big Data Analytics are essential to understand the unique profiles, which are being sourced in real time from sensor feeds and elderly people's data profiles. These Big Data source feeds can then be analyzed to provide analytics using machine learning to provide information on wellbeing and notification to social care personnel for monitoring and control via a dashboard.

A variety of processes and methods are available to support the analysis of Big Data, including information extraction, text analytics, audio

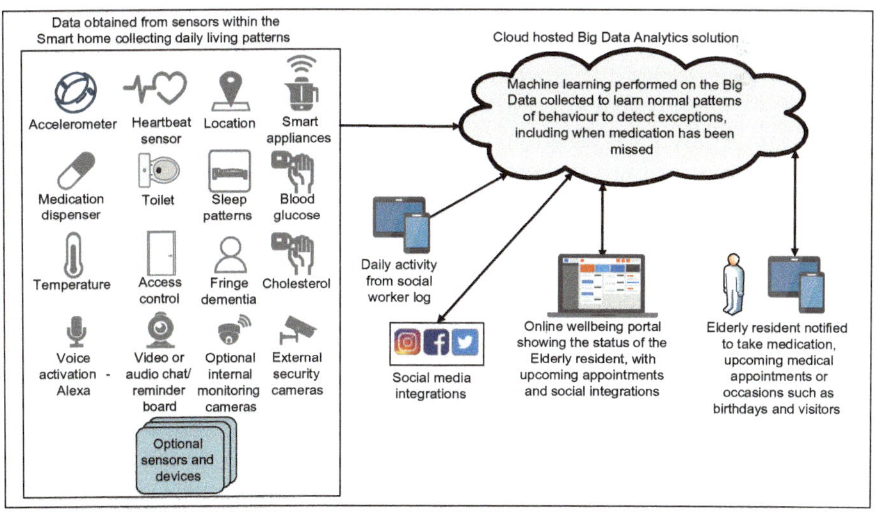

FIG 8.3 Data source feeds for Big Data Analytics using machine learning for wellbeing and social care notification and pre-emptive support to elderly residents.

analytics, and video analytics. The ability to extract insight from unstructured data through the process of information extraction is one of the factors that differentiates Big Data Analytics from traditional business intelligence. Adnan and Akbar [79] define information extraction as the process of extracting structured information from unstructured data in the form of entities, relations, objects, events, and other types. Text analytics refers to the range of techniques that extract information from textual data contained in sources including social network feeds, emails, blogs, online forums, surveys, documents, and call center logs [41]. Sentiment analysis is the process of identifying emotional states including sentiment, affect, and subjectivity from online texts [80]. Audio analytics are the techniques used to extract information from unstructured audio data, with its current primary use in call centers and in healthcare [81]. Gandomi and Haider [41] state that audio analytics are also referred to as speech analytics of which there are two technological approaches: large-vocabulary continuous speech recognition (LVCSR) and the phonetic-based approach. Video analytics refer to the techniques used to monitor, analyze, and extract insights from video streams, for example fall detection facilitated through the implementation of 2D and 3D video cameras in the home [82]; however, the key challenge is the size of the data [41].

Social media analytics refers to the analysis of structured and unstructured data generated by social media which can include social networks, blogs, microblogs, social news, social bookmarking, media sharing, question-and-answer sites, and review sites [41]. There are a variety of techniques for analysis, which include: modeling, sentiment analysis, social network analysis, and text mining [83]. The Home and Community Care Platform can integrate with social media platforms including Facebook and Twitter for the purposes of strengthening social bonds and monitoring the elderly, for example when an elderly resident's social media activity changes, caregivers can intervene accordingly [84].

Big Data Analytics is essential to the analysis of data from Smart homes. If large volumes of Big Data are being collected by care providers, a range of Big Data Analytics could be utilized. One example is Predictive analytics. Manogaran et al. [85] proposed a new architecture for collecting Big Data from IoT healthcare sensors, the Meta Fog-Redirection. The data collected include heart rate, body temperature, blood pressure, and blood glucose levels. The architecture consists of three phases: data collection, data transfer, and Big Data storage. When a reading from a sensor is detected which exceeds normal values, an alert is transmitted to a doctor. The proposed solution also uses the: "*stochastic gradient descent algorithm with logistic regression for developing the prediction model for heart disease*" [85, p. 385], therefore the system utilizes predictive analytics to identify if a patient has contracted heart disease. This example demonstrates how Big Data could be collected from Smart homes and analyzed to identify when medical intervention is required. Therefore, similar predictive or prescriptive analytics could be utilized for the purposes of enabling geriatric rehabilitation.

There are many benefits of Big Data Analytics reported in the literature, with usage ranging from large multinational companies to SMEs. Ram, Zhang, and Koronios [86, p. 223] report that Big Data Analytics can assist firms to: "*better exploit big data for improving customer satisfaction, managing supply chain risk, generating competitive intelligence, providing business real-time insights to help make important decisions and optimizing pricing if appropriately utilized.*" Wielki [87] claims that the key value of Big Data platforms is to accelerate the time it takes to make decisions, giving organizations answers to questions in seconds rather than months. Ahmed et al. [88] state that one of the benefits the IoT environment has provided is the ability to extract valuable information from users, allowing the prediction of future trends, and supporting fraud detection. The Home and Community Care Platform in Singapore supports ageing-in-place (the provision of care in the homes and community of the elderly) by ingesting and integrating data from a variety of heterogeneous data sources including discrete, unobtrusive sensors found in Smart homes, survey responses, wearable devices, and health records [84]. The platform provides real-time event processing to generate notifications, alerts, and escalations to enabling responsive delivery of care to elderly residents who require assistance, allowing healthcare professionals to rapidly respond when an elderly resident requires assistance. The platform utilizes advanced anomaly detection algorithms, predictive analytics, and deep diagnostics of daily living activities to provide care which surpasses the capabilities of traditional caregiving practices [84]. IoT and enabling technologies including cloud computing have facilitated the removal of data silos as traditionally data were only considered useful for the domain where the data originated; however, Big Datasets can now be combined.

Big Data Analytics is the evolution of Business Intelligence, providing the capability to analyze potentially enormous datasets of over 2TB, generated at a rapid pace and stored in a variety of structured, semistructured, and unstructured formats. It is anticipated that as the volumes of data generated globally continue to increase, the requirement to adopt Big Data Analytics will become more important, particularly in relation to Smart home monitoring for elderly people.

There are many use cases of how Big Data Analytics can support AAL. Goonawardene et al. [84] state that the Home and Community Care Platform will have the ability to integrate and manage potentially billions of sensors and related IoT devices; therefore Big Data Analytics are not only required for the analysis of healthcare data but additionally the statuses of sensors, battery replacement schedules, downtime alerts, and predictive maintenance, thus requiring minimal human supervision. The platform also aims to support sensors from any vendor or manufacturer and integrate with other IoT cloud platforms including Google Fit and Microsoft Health, providing further opportunities for further data collection and analysis. Therefore, Big Data Analytics can help healthcare platforms and diverse technology ecosystems to manage themselves.

There are many case studies of multinational firms that have successfully adopted Big Data Analytics. Danziger [89] outlines how Amazon utilizes Big Data Analytics to thrive in e-commerce. They implement dynamic pricing to change the price of products multiple times a day, making 2.5 million price changes daily, utilizing inventory data and competitors pricing. Amazon also screens purchases and return requests to detect fraudulent activity, recommends products to customers based on their activity and manages their distribution centers (stock control and alert workers when they are slow). Dallemand [90] provides a case study of how Marriott International have adopted Big Data Analytics to stay ahead of its competitors in a very competitive market, with new threats emerging such as community-based online platforms including Airbnb. Marriott are one of the largest hotel chains worldwide, operating in over 130 countries and continue expand by acquiring smaller brands. They use Big Data Analytics to monitor competitors' hotels and brands, set dynamic pricing, identify new revenue streams, and ensure that they maintain customer satisfaction, therefore achieving a completive advantage.

Vadillo et al. [6, p. 366] state that: "*Big Data offers new possibilities in the provision of healthcare services with added value in Smart homes. The processing of large amounts of data from multiple users and homes can improve the detection of potential risk events or help to prevent them, and even obtain common symptoms of early diseases.*" Therefore, the following section will discuss AAL and Smart homes.

8.5 Implementation of Big Data Analytics in a Smart home for geriatric rehabilitation

Monitoring solutions are currently available to allow families or carers to monitor the activity of relatives through a portal or App and receive alerts when specific events are detected. This is facilitated utilizing the data captured from a variety of discrete sensors placed. Some of the providers in the UK market include Canary Care [91], Howz [92], and Just Checking [93] which is designed for people with dementia. Alternatively, there are telehealthcare providers that provide a managed service by monitoring the activity of residents and contacting families when an event occurs or visit the property directly depending on the situation. UK Telehealthcare [94] provides a list of some telehealthcare providers in the United Kingdom. Telehealthcare providers that manage a large number of homes will require to store and process a large volume of data. It can be expected that as sensors technology increases to advance, more sensors are installed in homes, in addition to the increase in households adopting the technology, more data will be generated at a higher rate providing further challenges for telehealthcare providers.

Walsh [95 p. 54] outlines some of the challenges allowing elderly people to remain in their homes, one of which being the current Smart home solutions: *"The market for Smart home based solutions is nascent and often, the products have been developed for general-needs rather than specifically for the elderly. And of course, none of them accounted for the impact of COVID-19. A user-centered design approach to repurposing these tools would help drive adoption and impact."*

Big Data is expected to transform Smart homes and AAL delivery of services by: improving patient-centered services; diminishing costs; monitoring with real-time data analysis; and preventing potentially adverse events including side effect of medications, the early development of infections, and allergic reactions [96]. Zeadally et al. [9] suggest that Big Data Analytics and IoT can be utilized to improve Smart healthcare through the facilitation of evidence-based care. Big datasets can be aggregated from diverse sources, including IoT sensor data, which can then be analyzed to detect anomalies and appropriate treatments can be provided to patients. This suggests that Big Data Analytics would complement the AAL data captured through sensors in Smart homes.

The risk of falling is a major hazard to elderly people at home. Falls have been reported to cost around $8 billion per year and are the leading cause of accidental injury or death, accounting for 68% of hospital admissions for elderly patients [1]. Sarabia-Jacome et al. [97] proposed the utilization of predictive analytics and edge gateways for the use of fall detection to enrich the AAL environment. Predictive analytics have been utilized with cloud computing in fall detection; however, there are a number of potential issues with this approach including high bandwidth occupation, delay, low response times, security and privacy concerns. Using wearable technology, sensor data are captured and transmitted to a cloud computing platform, where the IoT Big Data is stored, and the deep learning process is undertaken. The local edge computing devices are then able to utilize the cloud-trained models to undertake predictive analytics on data captured from the sensors to identify if a fall has occurred more efficiently than a cloud-based model.

Sensor and Smart home technology are not restricted to the monitoring of events such as falls but can also be used proactively for early detection and improved monitoring of health conditions. Majumder et al. [98 p. 15] note that gait patterns can be used to indicate the early onset of some neurodegenerative diseases, such as Alzheimer's and Parkinson's and monitoring these patterns may provide useful diagnostic information. Basatneh, Najafi, and Armstrong [99] outline the potential of IoT devices to improve care for patients with diabetic foot ulcers or those at risk of developing a foot ulcer. Diabetes is the most common metabolic long-term health condition found in older people, with over 10% of people aged over

75 years in the United Kingdom and 14% aged over 85 years reported as diabetic [100] and it is estimated that around 10% of people with diabetes will develop a foot ulcer at some point, complications of which can potentially lead to amputation. Smart technologies include wearable devices to monitor the wound healing process; wearable technologies to enable continuous monitoring of health conditions including blood glucose monitoring devices; "Smart bathmats" that monitor foot temperatures to track the risk of foot ulceration; cardiovascular health monitoring systems; vital sign monitoring systems; and skin condition monitoring systems.

Another application of Big Data Analytics to support geriatric rehabilitation is the use of pressure sensors. The UK Dementia Directory [101] recommends bed, door, and chair sensor mats that can be installed into homes to alert a carer when an individual steps on a sensor mat, as it is common for individuals with dementia to wander at night. Therefore, if a care provider were monitoring a large number of residents, there is a large amount of sensor data that could be captured to be analyzed with Big Data Analytics technology to identify patterns for example when unexpected behavior occurs. There are a number of vendor tools available in the market for adaption to AAL including Google's Smart Analytics [102], Amazon Web Services Analytics [103], Zoho Analytics (Zoho [104]), the Microsoft Azure analytics platform [105], and Microsoft Power BI.

Fig. 8.4 shows how AAL technology and Big Data analytics can be integrated to give a proactive AAL health management system to support elderly people.

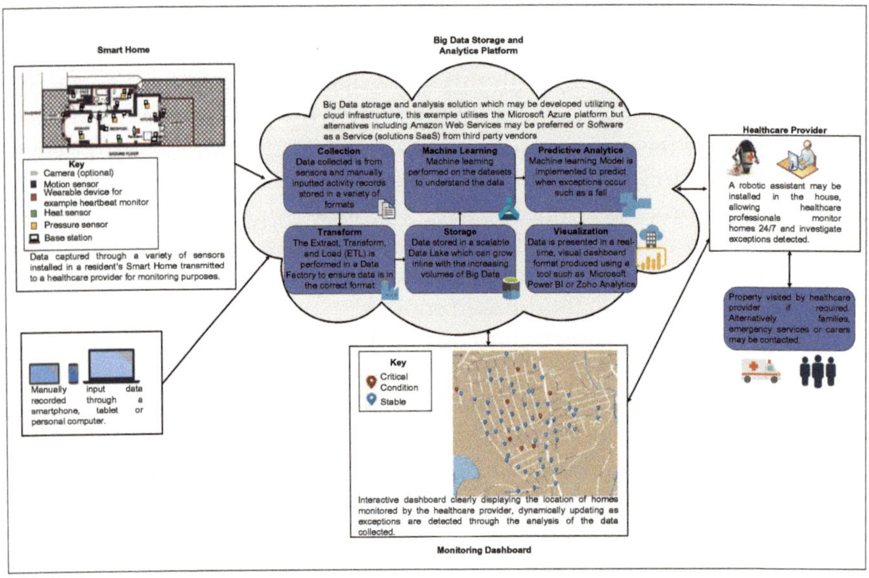

FIG. 8.4 Integration of AAL technology and Big Data Analytics to provide health management to elderly people.

There is potential for robot technology in Smart homes to further assist elderly people by integrating AAL to health systems where generic robots, which can be easily adapted to specialized tasks by physical "snap on" to perform for example cleaning duties or drug dispensing. Alternatively using "software changes" for example for improved social listening and conversation offer both physical and technology support to elderly people. The use of social media platforms such as Facebook provides a wider support network as elderly people tend to feel isolated [106] and this is particularly pertinent in the current COVID-19 climate. Agencies such as Age UK [107] offer local community support in terms of social gatherings for meals, hobbies, and entertainment. This concept could be expanded into a wider vision where the elderly people are linked via their Smart devices to other elderly people to provide a community network.

Anghel et al. [108], p. 2) state: "*Social robots may not only support older adults with daily activity, but at the same time they may contribute to emotional wellness by keeping older adults socially engaged and activating social interactions in communities. Moreover, they may not only drive the implementation of new services in various domains defined by WHO's age-friendly model in which older adults perceive the social robots as helpful companions, but they also promote the human-to-human interactions.*"

Big Data Analytics has the potential to improve the lives of elderly residents as healthcare providers can utilize the huge volumes of data that can be captured from Smart homes. For example, cameras can capture audio and video data, movement data can be captured from sensors and wearable devices or temperature data. It should be possible to retrofit these sensors to existing homes as outlined by Alsulami et al. [11]. As with the example proposed by Sarabia-Jacome et al. [97], Big Data Analytics can support deep learning to understand the patterns and behaviors of residents. When irregularities occur, alerts can be sent via text message or email to next of kin. If there is a delay in the recipient of the message responding, healthcare providers or emergency services can be notified. It has been reported that elderly people have died of coronavirus at home and have not been found for up to 2 weeks later [109], something which could be avoided by using this notification technology. The lack of sufficient geriatric accommodation particularly in major cities such as London where property cost can be £6,000 to £10,000 per m^2 (Wimbledon Park area) is resulting in increasing roof/loft and basement conversions in family homes increasing floor area by typically 30% to 45% subject to planning permission. This has the benefit of providing independent living accommodation with ground floor living for the elderly and the upper two floors can be used by the children/relatives to live in extended family units. This helps to ease the building pressure in inner cities and provides environmentally sourced floor area by repurposing and enlarging the existing family accommodation. This allows the next-generation access to property ownership and provides support to

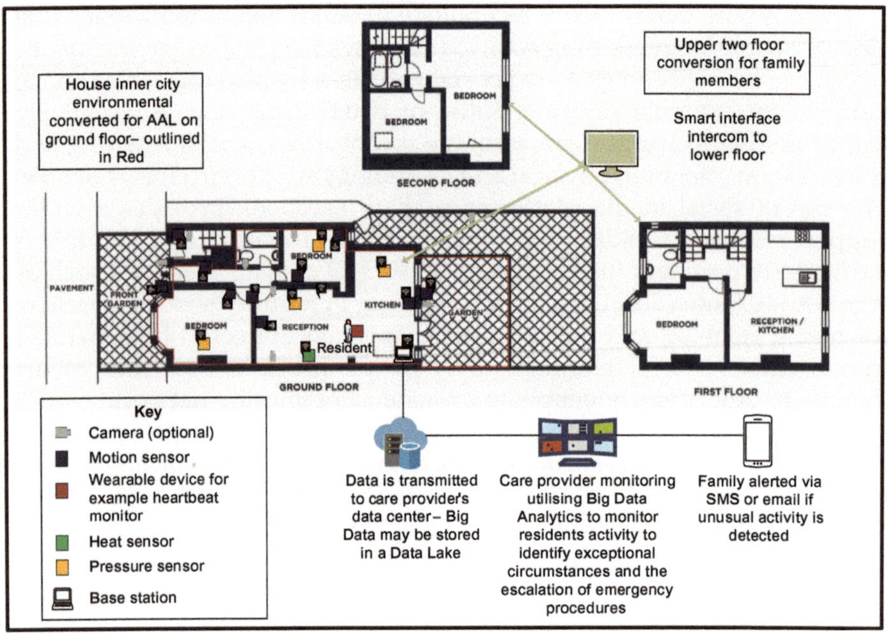

FIG. 8.5 House conversion for lower floor AAL and upper floors for family members, for example in London/major cities.

ageing family members to live independently in a supportive environment.

Fig. 8.5 shows a floor plan for modifying a family home and how AAL sensors can be installed to facilitate geriatric rehabilitation.

8.6 Conclusions

The increase in the numbers of elderly people means there is an increased pressure on local governments to provide high-quality care and service to citizens. At the same time, there is an increased demand for services to support independent living. The development of new purpose-built accommodation and the retrofitting of existing family homes to meet the needs will present a major challenge. It is expected that all IoT sensors embedded within a Smart home will have a specified lifespan, therefore they will likely need to be maintained and at some stage replaced, adding further financial implications.

Smart homes can generate enormous volumes of structured and unstructured Big Data from the various sensors and appliances embedded within the Smart home devices, including video files from cameras and movement data from wearable, infrared or pressure sensors. Deep learning techniques can be used with the data and predictive analytics can be performed on data as it is captured, allowing relatives or emergency services to be contacted if unusual behavior is detected. Residents' health can be monitored remotely, which may reduce the need for them to relocate to care homes. If a healthcare provider is monitoring a community of Smart homes, it will be essential for them to adopt Big Data Analytics. Fall detection is one example of how Big Data Analytics can be utilized for Smart homes to assist AAL but there are many other existing and potential applications to support the proactive use of AAL. The future use of robots, particularly in conversation and listening, is pertinent to Big Data Analytics integrated with deep learning algorithms in assessing mental health wellbeing and social care support training to assist elderly people in their home environment.

References

[1] J. Bennett, O. Rokas, L. Chen, Healthcare in the smart home: a study of past, present and future, Sustainability 9 (5) (2017) 840, doi:10.3390/su9050840.

[2] A. Yassine, et al., IoT big data analytics for smart homes with fog and cloud computing, Future Gener. Comput. Syst. 91 (2019) 563–573, doi:10.1016/j.future.2018.08.040.

[3] R. Maskeliunas, R. Damaševicius, S. Segal, A review of internet of things technologies for ambient assisted living environments, Future Internet (2019) 259, doi:10.3390/FI11120259.

[4] Boston Working Group, Boston working group on improving health care outcomes through geriatric rehabilitation. In: Medical care, Med Care, 1997, doi:10.1097/00005650-199706001-00003.

[5] Office of National Statistics (2019) Estimates of the very old, including centenarians, UK - Office for National Statistics. https://www.ons.gov.uk/peoplepopulationandcommunity/birthsdeathsandmarriages/ageing/bulletins/estimatesoftheveryoldincludingcentenarians/2002to2018 (Accessed 17 June 2020).

[6] L. Vadillo, et al., The role of smart homes in intelligent homecare and healthcare environments. In: Ambient Assisted Living and Enhanced Living Environments: Principles, Technologies and Control, 2016 345–394, doi:10.1016/B978-0-12-805195-5.00014-4.

[7] A. Margara, T. Rabl, Definition of data streams. In: Encyclopedia of Big Data Technologies, 2018 1–4, doi:10.1007/978-3-319-63962-8_188-1.

[8] M. Marjani, et al., Big IoT data analytics: architecture, opportunities, and open research challenges, IEEE Access. 5 (2017) 5247–5261, doi:10.1109/ACCESS.2017.2689040.

[9] S. Zeadally, et al., Smart healthcare, PSU Res. Rev (2019), doi:10.1108/prr-08-2019-0027.

[10] The European ambient assisted living innovation platform. In: Ambient Assisted Living Roadmap, Electronics, 2009 www.martinmanser.com Accessed 18 June 2020.

[11] Alsulami, M. et al. (2017) An enhanced conceptual model for using ambient assisted living to provide a home proactive monitoring system for elderly Saudi Arabians. doi: 10.1109/AICCSA.2017.214.

[12] Alsulami, M. and Atkins, A. (2016a) Elderly Saudi Arabians' perceptions and attitudes towards using ambient assisted living technologies. doi: 10.13140/RG.2.1.3170.5209.

[13] C. Wilson, T. Hargreaves, R. Hauxwell-Baldwin, Benefits and risks of smart home technologies, Energy Policy, 103, 2017 72–83, doi:10.1016/j.enpol.2016.12.047.

[14] M.Z. Uddin, W. Khaksar, J. Torresen, Ambient sensors for elderly care and independent living: a survey. In: Sensors (Switzerland), 2018, doi:10.3390/s18072027.
[15] D. Choi, H. Choi, D Shon, Future changes to smart home based on AAL healthcare service, J. Asian Architect. Build. Eng. 18 (3) (2019) 190–199, doi:10.1080/13467581.2019.1617718.
[16] Alsulami, M. and Atkins, A. (2016b) 'Factors influencing ageing population for adopting ambient assisted living technologies in the Kingdom of Saudi Arabia', Ageing Int., 41, pp. 227–239. doi:10.1007/s12126-016-9246-6.
[17] Alsulami, M., Atkins, A. and Campion, R. (2016) The use of smart watches to monitor heart rates in elderly people: a complementary approach. doi:10.1109/AICCSA.2016.7945809.
[18] Age UK (2019) Housing design, adaptations and support https://www.ageuk.org.uk/globalassets/age-uk/documents/policy-positions/housing-and-homes/ppp_housing_design_england.pdf (Accessed 8 October 2020).
[19] Which (2020) Getting a Needs Assessment for the Elderly - Which? https://www.which.co.uk/later-life-care/carers-and-caring/needs-assessment/getting-a-needs-assessment-af55g5x4xhf0 (Accessed 8 October 2020).
[20] Piddington, J. et al. (2020) The Housing Stock of The United Kingdom. www.bretrust.org.uk (Accessed 7 July 2020).
[21] F. Meijer, H. Visscher, L. Sheridan, Building regulations in Europe Part I: A comparison of the systems of building control in eight European countries, Housing and Urban and Policy Studies 23, England, United Kingdom, 2014.
[22] National House Building Council (NHBC) (2020a) 1.4 million new homes registered to be built in the past decade,reports NHBC. http://www.nhbc.co.uk/media-centre/articles/statistics/annual-statistics-2019/ (Accessed 1 July 2020).
[23] Ministry of Housing Communities and Local Government (2020) Dwelling Stock Estimates: 31 March 2019, England. https://assets.publishing.service.gov.uk/government/uploads/system/uploads/attachment_data/file/886251/Dwelling_Stock_Estimates_31_March_2019_England.pdf.
[24] National House Building Council (NHBC) (2020b) New home statistics review 2019.
[25] Natural Resources Canada (2020) Residential Sector Canada Table 21: Housing Stock by Building Type and Vintage Natural Resources Canada. https://oee.nrcan.gc.ca/corporate/statistics/neud/dpa/showTable.cfm?type=CP&sector=res&juris=ca&rn=21&page=5 (Accessed 30 September 2020).
[26] J. Rafferty, et al., From activity recognition to intention recognition for assisted living within smart Homes, IEEE Trans. Hum-Machine Syst 47 (3) (2017) 368–379, doi:10.1109/THMS.2016.2641388.
[27] M. Moore, Your smart home devices could all be about to stop working - here's why, TechRadar (2020). https://www.techradar.com/uk/news/your-smart-home-devices-could-all-be-about-to-stop-working-heres-why (Accessed 1 July 2020).
[28] Marr, B. (2020) The 5 Biggest Smart Home Trends In 2020, Forbes. https://www.forbes.com/sites/bernardmarr/2020/01/13/the-5-biggest-smart-home-trends-in-2020/#12939316389b (Accessed 1 July 2020).
[29] Kavanagh, S. (2020) How fast is 5G, 5G.co.uk. https://5g.co.uk/guides/how-fast-is-5g/ (Accessed 6 July 2020).
[30] R. Kitchin, Big data and human geography: opportunities, challenges and risks, Dialogues Hum. Geogr. 3 (2013) 262–267, doi:10.1177/2043820613513388.
[31] IDC (2019) Global DataSphere, IDC. https://www.idc.com/getdoc.jsp?containerId=IDC_P38353 (Accessed 15 December 2019).
[32] Coughlin, T. (2018) 175 Zettabytes By 2025, Forbes. https://www.forbes.com/sites/tomcoughlin/2018/11/27/175-zettabytes-by-2025/#52b570415459 (Accessed 15 December 2019).
[33] Marr, B. (2019) How Much Data Is There In the World? https://www.bernardmarr.com/default.asp?contentID=1846 (Accessed 15 December 2019).

[34] M. Blosch, J. Fenn, Understanding Gartner's Hype Cycles, Gartner (2018). https://www.gartner.com/doc/3887767 (Accessed 21 January 2020).
[35] H.E. Pence, What is Big Data and why is it important?, J. Educ. Technol. Syst 43 (2) (2015) 159–171, doi:10.2190/ET.43.2.d.
[36] P. Russom, Big data analytics, TDWI Best Practices Report, Fourth Quarter 19 (4) (2011) 1–34.
[37] Whishworks (2019) The State of Big Data in the UK 2019. www.whishworks.com (Accessed 27 October 2019).
[38] Bianchini, M. and Michalkova, V. (2019) OECD SME and Entrepreneurship Papers No. 15 Data Analytics in SMEs: Trends and Policies. doi: 10.1787/1de6c6a7-en.
[39] R. Kitchin, G. McArdle, What makes Big Data, Big Data? Exploring the ontological characteristics of 26 datasets, Big Data Soc 3 (1) (2016) 205395171663113, doi:10.1177/2053951716631130.
[40] Sicular, S. (2013) Gartner's Big Data Definition Consists of Three Parts, Not to Be Confused with Three 'V's, Forbes. http://www.forbes.com/sites/gartnergroup/2013/03/27/gartners-big-data-definition-consists-of-three-parts-not-to-be-confused-with-three-vs/ (Accessed 21 January 2020).
[41] A. Gandomi, M. Haider, Beyond the hype: Big data concepts, methods, and analytics, Int. J. Inf. Manage 35 (2) (2015) 137–144, doi:10.1016/j.ijinfomgt.2014.10.007.
[42] I. Lee, Big data: dimensions, evolution, impacts, and challenges, Business Horizons 60 (3) (2017) 293–303, doi:10.1016/j.bushor.2017.01.004.
[43] Rouse, M. (2020) What is a Zettabyte?, TechTarget. https://searchstorage.techtarget.com/definition/zettabyte (Accessed 17 October 2020).
[44] C. Olszak, M. Mach-Król, A conceptual framework for assessing an organization's readiness to adopt Big Data, Sustainability 10 (10) (2018) 3734, doi:10.3390/su10103734.
[45] N. Kshetri, The emerging role of Big Data in key development issues: opportunities, challenges, and concerns, Big Data Soc. 1 (2) (2014), doi:10.1177/2053951714564227.
[46] M. Willetts, A.S. Atkins, C. Stanier, A strategic Big Data analytics framework to provide opportunities for SMEs, Proc. 14th International Technology, Education and Development Conference, 2020 3033–3042, doi:10.21125/inted.2020.0893.
[47] Biehn, N. (2013) The Missing V's in Big Data: Viability and Value | WIRED. https://www.wired.com/insights/2013/05/the-missing-vs-in-big-data-viability-and-value/ (Accessed 15 November 2019).
[48] U. Sivarajah, et al., Critical analysis of Big Data challenges and analytical methods, J. Bus. Res 70 (2017) 263–286, doi:10.1016/J.JBUSRES.2016.08.001.
[49] M.A.U.D. Khan, M.F. Uddin, N Gupta, Seven V's of Big Data understanding Big Data to extract value, Proc. Zone 1 Conference of the American Society for Engineering Education - 'Engineering Education: Industry Involvement and Interdisciplinary Trends', ASEE Zone 1 2014, IEEE Computer Society, 2014, doi:10.1109/ASEEZone1.2014.6820689.
[50] A. Abbasi, S. Sarker, R.H.L Chiang, Big data research in information systems: toward an inclusive research agenda, J. Assoc. Inform. Syst, 17, 2016 i–xxxii. http://ezproxy.staffs.ac.uk/login?url=http://search.ebscohost.com/login.aspx?direct=true&db=bth&AN=113533298&site=ehost-live.
[51] Oracle (no date) What Is Big Data? https://www.oracle.com/uk/big-data/guide/what-is-big-data.html#link3 (Accessed 27 October 2019).
[52] J. Andreu, et al., Big Data for health, IEEE J. Biomed. Health Inform. (2015) 19, doi:10.1109/JBHI.2015.2450362.
[53] J.J.J.M. Seddon, W.L Currie, A model for unpacking big data analytics in high-frequency trading, J. Bus. Res 70 (2017) 300–307, doi:10.1016/j.jbusres.2016.08.003.
[54] Owais, S. S. and Hussein, N. S. (2016) Extract Five Categories CPIVW from the 9V's Characteristics of the Big Data, IJACSA) International Journal of Advanced Computer Science and Applications. www.ijacsa.thesai.org (Accessed 28 November 2019).
[55] Firican, G. (2017) The 10 Vs of Big Data. https://tdwi.org/articles/2017/02/08/10-vs-of-big-data.aspx (Accessed 14 November 2019).

[56] A. Alsaig, V. Alagar, O. Ormandjieva, A Critical Analysis of the V-Model of Big Data, Proc. 17th IEEE International Conference on Trust, Security and Privacy in Computing and Communications and 12th IEEE International Conference on Big Data Science and Engineering, Trustcom/BigDataSE 2018, Institute of Electrical and Electronics Engineers Inc., 2018, pp. 1809–1813, doi:10.1109/TrustCom/BigDataSE.2018.00273.
[57] Shafer, T. (2017) The 42 V's of Big Data and Data Science, KDnuggets. https://www.kdnuggets.com/2017/04/42-vs-big-data-data-science.html (Accessed 5 December 2019).
[58] N. Khan, et al., The 51 V's of Big Data: Survey, technologies, characteristics, opportunities, issues and challenges, Proc. ACM International Conference Proceeding Series, 2019 19–24, doi:10.1145/3312614.3312623.
[59] F. Amalina, et al., Blending big data analytics: review on challenges and a recent study, IEEE Access (2019) 1, doi:10.1109/ACCESS.2019.2923270.
[60] A. Gani, et al., A survey on indexing techniques for big data: taxonomy and performance evaluation, Knowl. Inform. Syst. 46 (2) (2016) 241–284, doi:10.1007/s10115-015-0830-y.
[61] A. Katal, M. Wazid, R.H. Goudar, Big data: issues, challenges, tools and good practices, Proc. 6th International Conference on Contemporary Computing, IC3 2013, 2013 404–409, doi:10.1109/IC3.2013.6612229.
[62] M.K. Saggi, S. Jain, A survey towards an integration of big data analytics to big insights for value-creation, Inf. Process. Manage 54 (5) (2018) 758–790, doi:10.1016/j.ipm.2018.01.010.
[63] A. De Mauro, M. Greco, M. Grimaldi, A formal definition of Big Data based on its essential features, Libr. Rev 65 (3) (2016) 122–135, doi:10.1108/LR-06-2015-0061.
[64] Statista (2019) Number of smartphone users worldwide from 2016 to 2021 (in billions), Statista. https://www.statista.com/statistics/330695/number-of-smartphone-users-worldwide/(Accessed 2 December 2019).
[65] C. Kimble, G. Milolidakis, Big Data and business intelligence: debunking the myths, Glob. Bus. Organ. Excell. 35 (1) (2015) 23–34 http://10.0.3.234/joe.21642.
[66] Laney, D., LeHong, D. and Lapkin, A. (2013) What Big Data Means for Business. at: https://www.ft.com/content/b1dec7f4-b686-11e2-93ba-00144feabdc0 (Accessed 4 November 2019).
[67] P. Tatum, S. Talebreza, J. Ross, Geriatric assessment: an office-based approach, Am. Fam. Physician 97 (2018) 776–784 784A.
[68] R.S. Kalan, M.O. Unalir, Leveraging big data technology for small and medium-sized enterprises (SMEs), Proc. 6th International Conference on Computer and Knowledge Engineering (ICCKE), IEEE, 2016, pp. 1–6, doi:10.1109/ICCKE.2016.7802106.
[69] C.-W.W. Tsai, et al., Big data analytics: a survey, J. Big Data 2 (1) (2015) 21, doi:10.1186/s40537-015-0030-3.
[70] P. Mikalef, et al., Big data analytics capabilities: a systematic literature review and research agenda, Inf. Syst. e-Bus. Manage 16 (3) (2018) 547–578, doi:10.1007/s10257-017-0362-y.
[71] P. Mikalef, et al., Big data analytics and firm performance: findings from a mixed-method approach, J. Bus. Res. 98 (2019) 261–276. https://doi.org/10.1016/j.jbusres.2019.01.044.
[72] M. Willetts, A.S. Atkins, C. Stanier, Barriers to SMEs adoption of Big Data analytics for competitive advantage, Proc. Fourth International Conference on Intelligent Computing in Data Sciences ICDS2020, Fez, Morocco, 2020.
[73] S.K. Song, et al., Prescriptive analytics system for improving research power, Proc. 16th IEEE International Conference on Computational Science and Engineering, CSE 2013, 2013, pp. 1144–1145, doi:10.1109/CSE.2013.169.
[74] V. Rajaraman, Big data analytics, Resonance 21 (8) (2016) 695–716, doi:10.1007/s12045-016-0376-7.

[75] P. Bihani, S.T. Patil, A comparative study of data analysis techniques, Int. J. Emerg.Trends Technol. Comput. Sci. 3 (2) (2014) 95–101. www.ijettcs.org (Accessed 1 December 2019).
[76] U. Sivarajah, et al., Role of big data and social media analytics for business to business sustainability: a participatory web context, Ind. Mark. Manage. (2019), doi:10.1016/j.indmarman.2019.04.005.
[77] K. Lepenioti, et al., Prescriptive analytics: literature review and research challenges, Int. J. Inform. Manag. 50 (2020) 57–70, doi:10.1016/j.ijinfomgt.2019.04.003.
[78] S. Kuttappa, Prescriptive analytics: The cure for a transforming healthcare industry, IBM, 2019. https://www.ibmbigdatahub.com/blog/prescriptive-analytics-cure-transforming-healthcare-industry (Accessed 1 December 2019).
[79] K. Adnan, R. Akbar, An analytical study of information extraction from unstructured and multidimensional big data, J. Big Data 6 (1) (2019), doi:10.1186/s40537-019-0254-8.
[80] Chen, Chiang and Storey, Business intelligence and analytics: from Big Data to big impact, MIS Quart. 36 (4) (2012) 1165, doi:10.2307/41703503.
[81] P. Vashisht, V. Gupta, Big data analytics techniques: a survey, Proc. International Conference on Green Computing and Internet of Things, ICGCIoT 2015, Institute of Electrical and Electronics Engineers Inc., 2016, pp. 264–269, doi:10.1109/ICGCIoT.2015.7380470.
[82] K. De Miguel, et al., Home camera-based fall detection system for the elderly, Sensors (Switzerland) 17 (12) (2017), doi:10.3390/s17122864.
[83] N.A. Ghani, et al., Social media big data analytics: a survey, Comput. Hum. Behav (2018), doi:10.1016/j.chb.2018.08.039.
[84] W.K.P.N.N.R. Goonawardene, et al., Technologies for ageing-in-place: The Singapore context. In: Living in Smart Cities: Innovation and Sustainability, 2018. https://ink.library.smu.edu.sg/sis_research/4242 (Accessed 16 October 2020).
[85] G. Manogaran, et al., A new architecture of Internet of Things and big data ecosystem for secured smart healthcare monitoring and alerting system, Future Gener. Comput. Syst. 82 (2018) 375–387, doi:10.1016/j.future.2017.10.045.
[86] J. Ram, C. Zhang, A. Koronios, The implications of Big Data Analytics on business intelligence: A qualitative study in China, Procedia Comput. Sci. 87 (2016) 221–226, doi:10.1016/J.PROCS.2016.05.152 Elsevier.
[87] J. Wielki, Implementation of the Big Data concept in organizations – Possibilities, impediments and challenges, Proc. Federated Conference on Computer Science and Information Systems, 2013, doi:10.1109/IC3.2013.6612229.
[88] E. Ahmed, et al., The role of big data analytics in Internet of Things, Comput. Netw. 129 (2017) 459–471, doi:10.1016/J.COMNET.2017.06.013.
[89] Danziger, C. (2019) How Amazon Used Big Data to Rule E-Commerce - insideBIGDATA, insideBigData. at: https://insidebigdata.com/2019/11/30/how-amazon-used-big-data-to-rule-e-commerce/ (Accessed 5 December 2019).
[90] Dallemand, J. (2019) What makes Marriott the big data Analytics Leader in Hospitality? [Case study], Datumize. https://blog.datumize.com/big-data-analytics-in-hospitality-marriott-international-case-study#smooth-scroll-top (Accessed 5 December 2019).
[91] Canary Care (2020) How the Canary Care Elderly Home Monitoring System Helps - Canary Care Global Ltd. https://www.canarycare.co.uk/how-it-helps/(Accessed 8 October 2020).
[92] Howz (2020) Howz Howz smart Monitoring System - Supporting Independent Living. at: https://howz.com/ (Accessed 8 October 2020).
[93] Just Checking (2020) Detailed activity monitoring, helping people stay at home for longer. https://justchecking.co.uk/ (Accessed 8 October 2020).
[94] UKTelehealthcare (2020) Local Providers – UKTelehealthcare – Telecare, Telehealth and TECS Hub. https://www.uktelehealthcare.com/local-providers/ (Accessed 8 October 2020).

[95] E. Walsh, Homes for Healthy Ageing: The Role of Innovation, Localis, 2020.
[96] V. Vimarlund, S. Wass, Big Data, Smart Homes and ambient assisted living. In: Yearbook of Medical Informatics, Thieme Medical Publishers, 2014, pp. 143–149, doi:10.15265/IY-2014-0011.
[97] D. Sarabia-Jacome, et al., Efficient deployment of predictive analytics in edge gateways: fall detection scenario, Proc. IEEE 5th World Forum on Internet of Things, WF-IoT 2019 - Conference Proceedings, Institute of Electrical and Electronics Engineers Inc., 2019, pp. 41–46, doi:10.1109/WF-IoT.2019.8767231.
[98] S. Majumder, et al., Smart homes for elderly healthcare—recent advances and research challenges, Sensors (Switzerland) (2017), doi:10.3390/s17112496.
[99] R. Basatneh, B. Najafi, D.G. Armstrong, Health sensors, smart home devices, and the internet of medical things: an opportunity for dramatic improvement in care for the lower extremity complications of diabetes, J. Diabetes Sci. Technol. 12 (3) (2018) 577–586, doi:10.1177/1932296818768618.
[100] British Geriatrics Society (2018) Diabetes British Geriatrics Society. https://www.bgs.org.uk/resources/diabetes (Accessed 9 October 2020).
[101] UK Dementia Directory (2020) Bed Leaving Sensor Mat Reviews. Best-Selling Alarm Mats for dementia. https://www.dementia.co.uk/products/bed-leaving-sensor-mat-alarm-mat (Accessed 2 October 2020).
[102] Google (2020) Smart Analytics Google Cloud. https://cloud.google.com/solutions/smart-analytics (Accessed 12 October 2020).
[103] Amazon Web Services (2020) Data Lakes and Analytics on AWS - Amazon Web Services. https://aws.amazon.com/big-data/datalakes-and-analytics/ (Accessed 12 October 2020).
[104] Zoho Corporation (2020) Self-service BI & Analytics Software – Zoho Analytics. https://www.zoho.com/analytics/ (Accessed 12 October 2020).
[105] Microsoft (2020) Azure Stream Analytics, Microsoft Azure. https://azure.microsoft.com/en-us/services/stream-analytics/(Accessed 12 October 2020).
[106] B. Wu, Social isolation and loneliness among older adults in the context of COVID-19: a global challenge, Glob. Health Res. Policy 5 (1) (2020), doi:10.1186/s41256-020-00154-3.
[107] Age UK (2020) Age UK. https://www.ageuk.org.uk/ (Accessed 17 June 2020).
[108] I. Anghel, et al., Smart environments and social robots for age-friendly integrated care services, Int. J. Environ. Res. Pub. Health 17 (2020) 3801, doi:10.3390/ijerph17113801.
[109] A. Wynne, Elderly people are dying alone at home due to coronavirus, Daily Mail Online, 2020. https://www.dailymail.co.uk/news/article-8397425/Elderly-people-dying-home-coronavirus.html (Accessed 28 June 2020).
[110] World Health Organization (2018) Ageing and health. https://www.who.int/news-room/fact-sheets/detail/ageing-and-health (Accessed 18 June 2020).

CHAPTER

9

Conclusion and perspectives

Mohamed-Amine Choukou[a], *Shabbir Syed-Abdul*[b]

[a]College of Rehabilitation Sciences; Centre on Aging, University of Manitoba, Winnipeg, Manitoba, Canada; Riverview Health Centre, Winnipeg, Manitoba, Canada, [b]Graduate Institute of Biomedical Informatics, Adjunct Professor at School of Gerontology Health Management, Taipei Medical University, Taipei, Taiwan

The goal of "Smart Home Technologies and Services for Geriatric Rehabilitation" was to address the roles and contributions of smart home technologies and services in supporting geriatric rehabilitation and to discuss the challenges of current practice and future innovation, especially with wireless technology and 5G advancements. The topics discussed in this book became even more interesting to disseminate just when we were writing the book as the COVID-19 pandemic created a burning platform for digital health and virtual care. The book provided a series of chapters by authors from interdisciplinary backgrounds and perspectives including technologists, clinicians, and health researchers, all supporting the "smart home movement."

Dr. Ganapathy provided an introduction with an exhaustive presentation of the smart home technologies and services for geriatric rehabilitation to initiate new comers to the field to existing technology-based approaches and presented them as the "new norm" moving forward. "Being more fit, active, mobile, safe, connected, independent, and self-reliant with an excellent quality of life will be the new mantra." Embracing smart home technologies poses new challenges in terms of training and professional development of healthcare providers. Dr. Mieronkoski et al. discussed the potential, benefits, and challenges with the use of the Internet of Things (IoT) based systems from a transdisciplinary health professionals' perspective. They concluded that the majority of current IoT-based systems are in an early stage of maturity and provided guidelines for the future implementation. Dr. Mieronkoski et al. emphasized the need for healthcare providers training in more integrative structures

DOI: https://doi.org/10.1016/B978-0-32-385173-2.00002-3

to support in-service education and transdisciplinary collaboration, as well as clear guidelines and regulations governing the use of Smart home technologies. Developing and implementing Smart home technologies need a strong involvement of older end-users to ensure appropriateness, cultural fit and usability. Dr. Alsulami et al. presented a conceptual Ambient Assisted Living Home Proactive Monitoring System (AALHPMS) to support elderly people in the Kingdom of Saudi Arabia (KSA) and the use of a web portal AgeinginKSA. The ambient assisted living (AAL) dashboard designed in the system allows the monitoring of older adults and track their activity in the real time, a first experience in the KSA. Dr. Edoh further discusses the design of a multidimensional smart home automation system to support long-term care at home in Germany, describing a system that goes beyond health, medical, and nursing care, and living assistance to include support for the caregivers.

The smart home applications listed above provide access to healthcare services that are not otherwise provided. In fact, telehealth enables healthcare professionals to screen, diagnose, provide consultation, treat, educate, rehabilitate, and monitor elderly patients. Telehealth can also empower elderly patients to be more independent at home. As such, the facilities provided by telehealth are essential for the provision of comprehensive and high-quality health care as people live longer with sometimes complex and chronic health needs. Dr. Alhuwail et al. provided and overview of different applications of telehealth to the care and rehabilitation of geriatric patients and discussed how leveraging them and integrating them into routine practice is a great opportunity to improve care quality and attain new levels of engagement with the elderly patients and their caregivers. There is a need for developing frameworks to strengthen the ongoing research and development work, and support the ongoing global "smart home movement."

Dr. Dorronzoro-Zubiete et al. described current smart home technologies reported in the scientific literature addressing cognitive health and have identified the frameworks proposed for designing these types of applications. They provided the readers with a list of evidence-based recommendations for designing smart home technologies and services for cognitive health of older adults. Some of the applications do not require the user to be active, while others do. This is the case of serious games for health which have attracted many industries and researchers due to their potential use in a wide scope of applications ranging from entertainment and exercising for adults to being used as an evaluation and training tool of cognitive or physical abilities. Dr. Muñoz et al. discussed the facilitators and barriers to the design, development, and evaluation of serious games for older adults as well as ideas for engaging with and accelerating development of this new and promising area. In particular, they emphasized the need of using reliable evaluation tools to provide greater evidence of the impact of serious games.

The objectives and modality of implementing smart home technologies and services, the topics such as Big Data and responsible data sharing and use are the first issues commonly and popularly discussed. Matthew Willetts et al. discussed Big Data, and the importance of Big Data analytics and its application to smart homes to support AAL for the purpose of geriatric rehabilitation. Several examples are provided throughout this chapter which highlight the benefits of this technology. The authors thoroughly explained how smart homes can generate enormous volumes of structured and unstructured Big Data from the various sensors and appliances embedded within the smart home devices, including video files from cameras and movement data from wearable, infrared, or pressure sensors. Matthew Willetts et al. emphasized how deep learning techniques can be used with the data and how predictive analytics can be performed on data as it is captured, allowing relatives or emergency services to be contacted if unusual behavior is detected.

In conclusion, this book presented a number of smart home applications for geriatric rehabilitation and discussed opportunities for creating more personalized and effective approaches. For many years to come, the "Smart home movement" is—and will be—an engaging field of research and development. We believe that the future is geared toward more technology-enabled (virtual) social interactions among older adults, their families, and healthcare providers. The future is also in the area of responsible and in-depth health telemonitoring and telepresence for both health and wellness.

Index

Page numbers followed by "*f*" and "*t*" indicate, figures and tables respectively.

FSC
www.fsc.org
MIX
Papier | Fördert
gute Waldnutzung
FSC® C083411

Kolibri 360 GmbH
Ferdinand-Jühlke-Straße 7
99095 Erfurt, Deutschland
produktsicherheit@kolibri360.de